SLIM FOR LIFE

Judith Wills

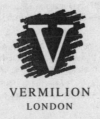

VERMILION
LONDON

WARNING

If you have a medical condition, or are pregnant, the diet and exercises described in this book should not be followed without first consulting your doctor. All guidelines and warnings should be read carefully and the author and publisher cannot accept responsibility for injuries or damage arising out of a failure to comply with the same.

1 3 5 7 9 10 8 6 4 2

Copyright © Judith Wills 1994

The right of Judith Wills to be identified as the Author of this book has been asserted by her in accordance with the Copyright, Designs and Patents Act, 1989.

First published in the United Kingdom in 1994 by Vermilion Arrow

This condensed edition published in 1999 by Vermilion an imprint of Ebury Press
Random House, 20 Vauxhall Bridge Road, London SW1V 2SA

Random House Australia (Pty) Limited
20 Alfred Street, Milsons Point, Sydney, New South Wales 2061, Australia

Random House New Zealand Limited
18 Poland Road, Glenfield, Auckland 10, New Zealand

Random House South Africa (Pty) Limited
Endulini, 5a Jubilee Road, Parktown 2193, South Africa

Random House UK Limited Reg. No. 954009

A CIP catalogue record for this book is available from the British Library

ISBN 0 09 940562 8

Designed by Roger Walker
Photography by Jon Stewart
Exercise clothing and trainers supplied by Nike

Printed and bound in Great Britain by
Caledonian International Book Manufacturing Ltd, Glasgow

CONTENTS

INTRODUCTION

Have you spent years 'on' and 'off' diets, but are now actually heavier than you were to start with?

Have you lost weight successfully, only to put it all back on again?

Have you tried to slim and failed because you couldn't stand either the diet food or the deprivation?

Are you completely disillusioned with the whole idea of dieting, but still you *hate* being overweight?

If you answered 'yes' to one or more of those questions, then you are one of ten million people in this country who are fat and fed up – and this is the book for you.

Slim for Life will become your friend, your helper, your confidante, your tutor. It's a guidebook that will lead you to success because it doesn't just tell you to 'eat less': it helps you to see why you've been eating too much and shows you how to control your intake.

Slim for Life takes you, step by logical step, through a unique, new, exciting – and, yes, challenging – self-help programme which will ensure that you become slim and *stay* slim once and for all.

In *Slim for Life* there are no gimmicks; no promises about exactly how much weight you will lose in a given space of time. There is no 'set', tyrannical diet in this book, no forbidden foods, no dubious regimes to follow – and few, if any, rules. Yet you *will* lose weight if you work through the six-step programme at your own pace and don't progress to the next step until you have mastered the one before. And you will *keep* the weight off.

Because *Slim for Life* is a book to get you *thinking* and *doing* rather than just a book to read, and because there *is* so much in it for you to absorb and do, you may take not hours, or even days, but weeks to work through its pages. But when you consider the umpteen hours you have wasted trying and failing on previous diets, or simply on feeling miserable and despising your own body, it will be time you can afford.

It will also be time you enjoy – yes, I am confident that for the first time you will actually *enjoy* a book that is helping you to lose weight!

CHAPTER ONE

Take a New Look at Food

Overweight people tell me time after time that they can't lose weight on a diet. They will tell me, say, that even though they are only eating 1,000 calories a day they aren't shedding an ounce.

Yet in every trial conducted where people were put in controlled conditions and fed 1,000 calories a day, they *all* lost weight. Lots of it. A recent report has backed up what I already knew: that very many would-be dieters eat and drink masses more than they think they are eating and drinking. The truth is that unless you know what you're doing it is possible to *appear* to be eating little when in fact you are eating quite a lot.

Old-style versus new-style eating

Here's an example of a typical day's 'hardly eating anything' that *won't result in the average woman losing any weight at all*.

Breakfast
Large glass fruit juice
Small helping (60 g, 2¼ oz) muesli with milk to cover

Lunch
Small piece (approx. 50 g, 2 oz) Cheddar
with 2 cream crackers very lightly buttered
1 tomato, little lettuce
1 fruit yogurt

Dinner
1 small lamb chop
1 small baked potato with small knob butter
Small portion mixed peas and carrots
Small portion (approx. 75 g, 3 oz) ice cream
topped with 2 teaspoons chopped mixed nuts

Throughout day
Coffee or tea with milk, no sugar

This is a day's consumption that, to the 'dieter', will seem very little on the plate, but in fact it is not only very high in fat and low in carbohydrates (the complete opposite of a good, long-term healthy diet) but also contains in the region of 1,900 calories – about the amount of calories an average woman taking little exercise will consume in an average day. If calorie intake equals calorie output, there will be no weight gain – but no loss, either!

And yet, eating like that, the consumer is under the impression she *is* dieting and feels cross that there are no results. *No* bread! *No* pastry! *No* chocolate! *No* alcohol! *No* sugar in her coffee! *No* fried foods! *No* between-meal snacks! She's been so good, she feels, by sticking to fruit juice, healthy muesli, crispbreads and small portions of everything.

One of the first keys to successful weight loss and weight maintenance is *knowledge*. The 'dieter' illustrated above lacks knowledge about the fat-rich foods.

These were her main mistakes that day:

- Using full-cream milk on cereal and in drinks.
- Muesli is denser than most cereals and contains more fat. Even a small bowlful will be much higher in calories than a larger helping of most other cereals.
- Cheddar cheese is a very high-fat food. Cream crackers are quite high in fat, too – and butter, even lightly spread, adds many more calories.

- Fruit yogurt can be low in fat and calories, but not always. Some contain whole milk, added sugar and even added cream.
- Lamb chops, unless very well trimmed, are a high-fat meat. Even grilling doesn't help a lot, unless you remove the visible fat.
- That small knob of butter on the potato could contain almost as many calories as the potato itself. Fats are easy to miscalculate as they are dense, high-calorie foods.
- Ice cream is a reasonable dessert but even a few nuts add on lots of fat and calories. Almost all nuts are very high in fat.

This is what I call the 'old-fashioned British' style of eating that has contributed towards our weight problem. With a bit more knowledge, this woman could halve the fat and calories in her day's eating *without* substantially changing the type of food she eats, *without* feeling hungry, and yet *with* more food actually on the plate and *with* between-meal snacks too. She will also be giving herself a much, much healthier diet as she slims down.

Here's that same day's eating converted at least partially to the 'new style' – the style we should aim for to get slim.

Breakfast
1 piece fresh fruit
Medium helping flaked cereal (any kind except with added sugar) with skimmed milk to cover

Mid-morning
1 banana

Lunch
40 g (1½ oz) half-fat Cheddar-style cheese
with 1 slice wholemeal bread with a little low-fat spread
Large salad
1 low-fat diet fruit yogurt

Dinner
1 small extra-lean lamb fillet steak, grilled
1 large baked potato topped with 2 teaspoons fromage frais
Large portion fresh peas
Large portion carrots
Medium portion reduced-fat ice cream
or ice cream substitute

Throughout day
Coffee or tea with skimmed milk

The new-style pyramid places a much greater emphasis on the natural (or nearly natural) high-carbohydrate foods: bread, potatoes, grains of all kinds – including rice – breakfast cereals and pasta. It places almost as much emphasis on fruits, dried fruits, vegetables and pulses. All these foods in the two groups are the 'complex carbohydrates' that together will form the bulk of your diet. (Pulses, by the way, are also high-protein foods, but for the purposes of our new-style pyramid they are best included with the two vegetable and starch groups.)

Our protein needs aren't great – about 10 to 15 per cent of calories in our total diet – so in keeping the meat, fish and dairy-produce part of the pyramid to 20 per cent of total calories and by retaining in this group only the reasonably low-fat items (such as white fish, poultry with no skin and the reduced-fat versions of milk and cheese), we ensure that in adding protein to the diet you are not by default adding too much extra fat. In this protein group I include the new vegetable-protein foods, such as TVP (soya protein), Quorn and tofu, all of which are reasonably low-fat sources of protein.

I estimate that at least 10 per cent of the calories in this food group will be fat calories; the other 10 per cent will be protein. (Protein is also present in the complex-carbohydrate group of foods; bread, rice and so on all have reasonable amounts and even fruit and vegetables have a little. So, in all, the new-style diet will easily meet protein needs.)

You can see from these pyramids how the two diets compare:

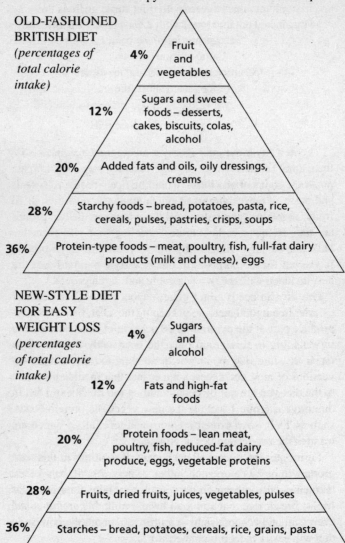

OLD-FASHIONED BRITISH DIET
(percentages of total calorie intake)

4% — Fruit and vegetables

12% — Sugars and sweet foods – desserts, cakes, biscuits, colas, alcohol

20% — Added fats and oils, oily dressings, creams

28% — Starchy foods – bread, potatoes, pasta, rice, cereals, pulses, pastries, crisps, soups

36% — Protein-type foods – meat, poultry, fish, full-fat dairy products (milk and cheese), eggs

NEW-STYLE DIET FOR EASY WEIGHT LOSS
(percentages of total calorie intake)

4% — Sugars and alcohol

12% — Fats and high-fat foods

20% — Protein foods – lean meat, poultry, fish, reduced-fat dairy produce, eggs, vegetable proteins

28% — Fruits, dried fruits, juices, vegetables, pulses

36% — Starches – bread, potatoes, cereals, rice, grains, pasta

Near the top of the new-style pyramid are the fats you add in recipes and at table; the very high-fat foods such as dressings and cream; and all the other high-fat foods featured lower down in the old-style diet but not in this pyramid, e.g., pastries and baked foods.

The tip of the new pyramid allows for sugars and alcohol. These last two groups at the top of the pyramid joined together amount to 16 per cent of the total calorie intake and compose the fatty, sugary foods we should be cutting down on.

THE EASIEST WAYS TO CUT FAT

- Make changes gradually.
- Make swops in what you buy.
- Make swops in how you cook.
- Alter the balance on your plate.
- Make changes you are most able to live with.
- Incorporate into your diet sensible amounts of what you can't live without.

Make changes gradually

Although the 'kill or cure' approach works for some people, usually the best method for change is 'little by little'. Also, as your digestive system takes time to adapt to a different diet, this makes sense physically as well as emotionally. And it makes sense in a third way: your palate will then painlessly adapt to what you offer it.

Here are a couple of examples of making changes gradually rather than quickly:

You decide to cut down on fat by using skimmed milk instead of whole milk. But your palate tells you you dislike the skimmed milk in your tea and on your cereals: it doesn't 'taste right'. So you go back to your whole milk. *What you should have done* was choose semi-skimmed milk as a compromise for a few weeks and then tried the fully skimmed.

You decide that one of the reasons your fat intake is high is your love of biscuits, so you determine to cut them out. But after a day or two you are craving biscuits, so you start eating them even more avidly than before. *What you should have done* was either replace your biscuits with a lower-fat, lower-calorie kind (if possible) or cut down the number (perhaps by buying them individually wrapped).

Make changes gradually so you have time to get accustomed to them in every way. After a time they are incorporated into your life as if they are habits you have always had.

Make swops in what you buy

Although it is the case that you are, largely (perhaps *very* largely!), what the food industry has made you, the good news is that if we show the food industry – through what we buy in the supermarkets – that what we want is lower fat, lower sugar, healthier produce, then eventually that message will get through and the shelves will reflect our wishes.

That means making a determined and wholesale effort to shop the new-style pyramid way. Since there is only profit to be made in manufacturing and selling packets of cream cakes or trifle mixes and the like if the products disappear from the shop shelves, any line that sits there for too long gets replaced by something that *will* sell.

Already all the supermarkets and most of the smaller shops are offering reduced-fat, reduced-sugar, reduced-calorie versions of high-fat, high-cal, high-sugar foods, yet still it is frequently more difficult for us to locate these lines than the traditional versions. However, the most popular of the reduced-fat items, the ones with which we are very familiar, are big sellers and are therefore stocked just as prominently as their counterparts, skimmed milk and reduced-fat spreads being the two that come to mind first.

The following are all swops that will save masses of fat calories. Tick all the swops that are new to you and try out one or two of them every time you do a shop.

☐ **Low-fat spread instead of butter/ordinary margarine**
Yes, low-fat spread is a high-fat food, but it contains only
half the fat (or less) of the conventional spreads and it tends
to spread thinner, too. If you have tried low-fat spread
before and not liked it, pick a small size of a different
brand, because taste quality varies enormously and some
are very pleasant indeed.

☐ **Low-fat yogurt instead of whole-milk yogurt**   Read the
labels to make sure that the yogurt you buy really is low in
fat; some aren't.

☐ **Lower-fat cheeses instead of traditional cheeses**   More
and more reduced-fat varieties, such as Cheddar, Edam,
Cheshire, Red Leicester, processed slices, soft cream-type
cheeses, cheese spreads, roulé and cottage, are available
and many of the traditional cheeses are lower in fat and
calories than other varieties. For instance, Brie and
Camembert have less fat and fewer calories (about 85 per
25 g, 1 oz) than cream cheese or Cambozola (110 per 25 g,
1 oz). Practise reading the labels and comparing the fat
contents of the various cheeses.

Cheddar addicts often don't like the reduced-fat imita-
tion varieties (again, some are better than others). If that
includes you, here are three tips: (1) the reduced-fat versions are fine in cooking, (2) if you buy a very strong Cheddar (e.g., mature farmhouse or extra mature) you will
probably find that half your normal amount suffices
because the strong varieties are much more flavoursome
than the mild Cheddars, and (3) grated cheese goes further.

☐ **Lean cuts of meat instead of the traditional cuts**   Due
to demand, leaner meat is being produced all the time, but
even so I still see a lot of very fatty cuts of meat in the
butchers' and supermarkets. Ignore those and always go for
the extra-lean cuts that are labelled as such. Many people

don't choose these because they are more expensive, but if you buy the cheaper cuts and then have to cut the fat off (or throw melted fat away after cooking) it is false economy. Not only that, but by buying the lean cuts you remove the temptation to eat the fat rather than throw it away.

You can get lean mince, lean trimmed chops, lean bacon, low-fat sausages and low-fat ham.

Tuna in brine instead of tuna in oil   Tuna in oil is a high-fat food; tuna in brine is a very low-fat food. If you like tuna it's an easy swop to make.

Straight-cut, thick-cut chips instead of crinkled chips or thin-cut chips   Crinkled and/or thin chips absorb much more fat than straight and thick-cut chips, so if you are a chip addict the fat- and calorie-saving can be great. Oven chips are a good bet, too; as brands vary, go for the ones that contain least fat.

Low-fat crisps instead of regular crisps   The saving per pack isn't much, but if you're very partial to crisps it could make a difference.

Spraying oil instead of cooking oil   You can now buy a special spray-on oil that gives the pan a very light coating for 'frying' without adding calories.

Extra-thick single cream or fromage frais or Greek-style yogurt instead of double cream.

'Alternative to cream' (half the fat) **or cream in an aerosol container** (because it contains so much air that a big 'squirt' works out at minimal calories) **instead of single cream.**

Lower-fat dressings instead of full-fat versions   These almost all taste fine, so swop full-fat mayonnaise for a reduced-calorie type. Salad cream, Thousand Island, tartare and French dressing are available in no- or low-cal versions.

☐ **Lower-fat proteins instead of high-fat proteins** Make the decision to base more main-course dishes on the lower-fat protein foods such as lean chicken, turkey, veal (if you will eat it), Quorn, white fish and pulses. Cod contains 8 per cent fat calories, while steak (without the fat border on it) has 32 per cent fat calories. So if you're a red-meat fan, say, decide to give up one red-meat meal a week to start with. Further on in this chapter you will find many ideas for making lower-fat meals just as interesting, tasty and satisfying as high-fat meals.

Make swops in how you cook

You can cut out even more fat from your cooking by using the following methods. Again, tick all those that are new to you and aim regularly to try out each one.

☐ **Dry-fry, don't deep-fry** Many things that you used to fry can nowadays be oven-baked, but, if you don't want to do that, the next best thing is to dry-fry. You need a good, heavy-bottomed, non-stick frying pan and a tiny brushing of oil (or the new spray-on oil). Once the pan is heated, many foods, from fish to sauté potatoes, can be cooked this way.

☐ **Grill fatty foods, don't fry them** You'll cut out even more fat calories if you grill, say, a slice of bacon over a slatted splash guard so that the fat in the meat melts, runs through the slats and is easy to discard. Grill foods such as bacon and sausages until really well done in order to eliminate even more fat.

☐ **Experiment with methods that reduce the fat or oil content in your favourite recipes** Many new-style recipes for you to try are included in Step Four, but almost any recipe can be adapted in a similar way. For instance, if you're browning onions or meat for a casserole, you could reduce the specified fat or oil down to nearly nothing, especially if you use non-stick cookware. Also, many soup recipes suggest frying the vegetables first in oil, but you can usually omit this step and simply simmer them in stock before blending.

☐ **If you're using mince in a recipe, pour off any fat that rises to the top** (or use a fat-absorbing brush to lift it off).

☐ **Casseroles can be made in advance,** left in the fridge and then any solid fat that appears on the top is easily removed.

☐ **Use reduced-fat cooking spread** for baking.

All these things are easy to do and won't detract from the taste of your cooking at all.

Alter the balance on your plate

Get into the habit of 'thinking pyramid' every time you make up a plateful of food for yourself. See how often you can compose a meal of which the largest part is complex carbohydrates from the base of the pyramid and the next largest is from the fruit and veg section, followed by a smaller-than-usual portion of your protein food and a little bit of something fatty.

Old-style balance Large steak or slices of roast meat; medium portion of potatoes; big knob of butter on both potatoes and steak; small portion of peas.

New-style balance Much smaller steak or slices of roast meat; much larger portion of potatoes; at least two helpings of vegetables; a very small knob of butter on the potatoes, and fat-free gravy over the rest of the plate to avoid dryness.

Keep looking back at that pyramid and get the balance right! *It will take time,* but don't worry about this.

You can alter the balance in other ways, too. Instead of that steak-and-potatoes meal, try one that is based on carbohydrates

– say, a big plate of spaghetti or rice topped with a vegetable stir-fry containing just a very *little* meat.

Make changes you are most able to live with

Some of the suggestions I make may seem more easy, more pleasant and more practical to you than others. Work first on the ones that seem easiest. Everyone is different; your diet doesn't have to be exactly the same as everyone else's. Your preferences matter. If you don't take account of them you won't succeed in losing weight and keeping it off. You're not being asked to sacrifice everything you hold dear, but only to look and see if there are ways of improving your diet and to understand that your taste in food can alter.

If, after giving something – say, low-fat spread – a fair trial, you just can't get on with it, well, don't worry, you don't *have* to eat low-fat spread to get slim.

*   *   *

'I've always had a sweet tooth, though. Isn't it sweet things rather than fat that are keeping me fat?'

Sweet tastes are something we are, literally, born to enjoy. Breast milk is sweet; so is formula milk. By the time we are weaned, the taste for sweet foods is well established. Both breast and formula milks also contain fat and it's this seductive combination of sugar and fat that is, I believe, the main problem.

Sugar, on its own, isn't irresistible. You can carry out a taste test similar to the one for fat described earlier. Place a sugar bowl in front of you and see how much of the sugar you can eat, by itself, before having to admit defeat. It won't be much. It's just too sweet! Nobody gets fat through a weakness for confectionery that doesn't contain fat – boiled sweets, for instance, or fruit pastilles. The sweet items that most people crave, and that give them a weight problem, are the fat-laden ones like chocolate (which we'll come to in a minute), cakes, biscuits, cheesecakes, pastries and creamy desserts.

In fact our national consumption of packet sugars – e.g. granulated – has halved in recent years. But, although increasing numbers of us are drinking tea and coffee without adding sugar and using less sugar on cereal, there has been a massive increase in our consumption of those hidden sugars in the items listed above.

We should try to reduce the amount of sugary foods that we eat for three main reasons:

1. The combination of fat and sugar in most sweet foods will make you eat even if you aren't hungry. You will be inclined to eat puddings, desserts and snacks which literally 'slip down' before you have really noticed.

2. Sugar, in all its forms – white, brown, glucose, syrup, fructose – contains carbohydrate but little else. Even honey and molasses contain very few other nutrients: no vitamins, no minerals, but approximately 100 calories per 25 g (1 oz). So if you eat a lot of the high-sugar items at the expense of more nutritious foods, your diet may lack vital nutrients.

3. Simple sugars, with the exception of fructose (fruit sugar), are not so effective in curbing hunger as are the complex carbohydrates. They are more quickly absorbed into the bloodstream, so, at first, you will feel full. But, as the sugar is so rapidly dealt with, this blood-glucose level quickly sinks, leaving you feeling hungry again soon.

However, for sweet-toothers, all is not lost! Although, as with fat, experiments have shown that it is possible to conquer a desire for sweet foods as quickly as it is to overcome a taste for fatty ones, you needn't go cold turkey and face another 'no sweet foods' tyrannical diet. That won't work for you. We can apply to sugar much of the advice I gave you for cutting down painlessly on fats.

Make changes gradually

If you do take sugar in tea or coffee and want to cut down, do so by a very small amount at a time. In a few weeks you may well be able to give up altogether. I know many people who used to take drinks sweetened and who now find the taste awful if sugar is added by mistake.

* * *

'I don't enjoy healthy foods so how can I diet?'
'I don't like salads or many vegetables.'

What people who say they don't like 'health foods' – particularly salads and vegetables – in my experience really mean is one of the following:

'I don't like certain things that appear to me to come under the category "health foods"' (e.g., brown rice, beansprouts, grapefruit, figs).

'I dislike certain vegetables and salads because I associate them with unappetising offerings in the past' (e.g., watery, overboiled greens and limp lettuce salads).

'I haven't tried many of these foods but I don't think I would like them'.

None of these feelings, when you examine them closely, actually mean that you won't like eating in a slimmer, more healthy way *if* you accept that some of your old ideas and prejudices may be wrong.

Look at the chart that follows. There are four lists of food items. Go down each list and tick which box in the columns alongside applies to you for every food.

List One

	Like	Will eat	Haven't tried	Dislike at present
White bread	☐	☐	☐	☐
Brown bread	☐	☐	☐	☐
Wholemeal bread	☐	☐	☐	☐
Rye bread	☐	☐	☐	☐
Speciality breads (e.g., Ciabatta)	☐	☐	☐	☐
Pitta	☐	☐	☐	☐
Crispbread	☐	☐	☐	☐
Crustini sticks	☐	☐	☐	☐
Grissini sticks	☐	☐	☐	☐
Baked potatoes	☐	☐	☐	☐
Boiled potatoes	☐	☐	☐	☐
Mashed potatoes	☐	☐	☐	☐
Sweet potatoes	☐	☐	☐	☐
Baked beans	☐	☐	☐	☐
Butter beans	☐	☐	☐	☐
Red kidney beans	☐	☐	☐	☐
Black-eye beans	☐	☐	☐	☐
Chick peas	☐	☐	☐	☐
Green lentils	☐	☐	☐	☐
Home-made lentil soup	☐	☐	☐	☐
Weetabix	☐	☐	☐	☐
Porridge	☐	☐	☐	☐
Bran flakes	☐	☐	☐	☐
Fruit 'n' Fibre	☐	☐	☐	☐

	Like	Will eat	Haven't tried	Dislike at present
Spaghetti	☐	☐	☐	☐
Tagliatelle	☐	☐	☐	☐
Lasagne	☐	☐	☐	☐
Brown rice	☐	☐	☐	☐
Long-grain rice	☐	☐	☐	☐
Wild rice	☐	☐	☐	☐
Couscous	☐	☐	☐	☐
Bulgar wheat	☐	☐	☐	☐
Buckwheat	☐	☐	☐	☐
Pancakes	☐	☐	☐	☐
Polenta	☐	☐	☐	☐
Noodles	☐	☐	☐	☐

List Two

	Like	Will eat	Haven't tried	Dislike at present
Apple	☐	☐	☐	☐
Apricots, fresh	☐	☐	☐	☐
Apricots, dried	☐	☐	☐	☐
Banana	☐	☐	☐	☐
Blackcurrants	☐	☐	☐	☐
Currants, dried	☐	☐	☐	☐
Cherries	☐	☐	☐	☐
Dates, fresh	☐	☐	☐	☐
Dates, dried	☐	☐	☐	☐
Gooseberries	☐	☐	☐	☐
Grapefruit, pink	☐	☐	☐	☐
Grapes	☐	☐	☐	☐

	Like	Will eat	Haven't tried	Dislike at present
Kiwifruit	☐	☐	☐	☐
Mango	☐	☐	☐	☐
Melon, water	☐	☐	☐	☐
Melon, ogen	☐	☐	☐	☐
Nectarine	☐	☐	☐	☐
Orange	☐	☐	☐	☐
Peaches, fresh	☐	☐	☐	☐
Peaches, dried	☐	☐	☐	☐
Pears, fresh	☐	☐	☐	☐
Pears, dried	☐	☐	☐	☐
Prunes, Californian	☐	☐	☐	☐
Prunes, stoned	☐	☐	☐	☐
Raspberries	☐	☐	☐	☐
Rhubarb	☐	☐	☐	☐
Satsuma	☐	☐	☐	☐
Strawberries	☐	☐	☐	☐

List Three

	Like	Will eat	Haven't tried	Dislike at present
Artichoke, Jerusalem	☐	☐	☐	☐
Artichoke hearts	☐	☐	☐	☐
Asparagus	☐	☐	☐	☐
Aubergine	☐	☐	☐	☐
Avocado	☐	☐	☐	☐
Beans, broad	☐	☐	☐	☐
Beans, French	☐	☐	☐	☐
Beans, runner	☐	☐	☐	☐

	Like	Will eat	Haven't tried	Dislike at present
Beansprouts	☐	☐	☐	☐
Beetroot	☐	☐	☐	☐
Broccoli	☐	☐	☐	☐
Brussels sprouts	☐	☐	☐	☐
Cabbage, green	☐	☐	☐	☐
Cabbage, red	☐	☐	☐	☐
Cabbage, white	☐	☐	☐	☐
Carrots	☐	☐	☐	☐
Cauliflower	☐	☐	☐	☐
Celery	☐	☐	☐	☐
Chinese leaves	☐	☐	☐	☐
Corn on the cob	☐	☐	☐	☐
Courgettes	☐	☐	☐	☐
Cucumber	☐	☐	☐	☐
Leek	☐	☐	☐	☐
Lettuce	☐	☐	☐	☐
Mushrooms	☐	☐	☐	☐
Onion, Spanish	☐	☐	☐	☐
Onion, spring	☐	☐	☐	☐
Onion, red	☐	☐	☐	☐
Parsnip	☐	☐	☐	☐
Peas, fresh	☐	☐	☐	☐
Peas, frozen	☐	☐	☐	☐
Pepper, green	☐	☐	☐	☐
Pepper, red	☐	☐	☐	☐

	Like	Will eat	Haven't tried	Dislike at present
Spinach, fresh	☐	☐	☐	☐
Swede	☐	☐	☐	☐
Sweetcorn	☐	☐	☐	☐
Tomato	☐	☐	☐	☐
Tomato, cherry	☐	☐	☐	☐
Watercress	☐	☐	☐	☐

List Four

	Like	Will eat	Haven't tried	Dislike at present
Low-fat soft cheese	☐	☐	☐	☐
Diet cottage cheese	☐	☐	☐	☐
Cod	☐	☐	☐	☐
Monkfish	☐	☐	☐	☐
Brill	☐	☐	☐	☐
Lemon sole	☐	☐	☐	☐
Trout, brown	☐	☐	☐	☐
Trout, rainbow	☐	☐	☐	☐
Tuna in brine	☐	☐	☐	☐
Salmon, fresh	☐	☐	☐	☐
Crabmeat	☐	☐	☐	☐
Mussels	☐	☐	☐	☐
Prawns	☐	☐	☐	☐
Scallops	☐	☐	☐	☐
Squid	☐	☐	☐	☐
Turkey	☐	☐	☐	☐
Venison	☐	☐	☐	☐
Quorn	☐	☐	☐	☐

	Like	Will eat	Haven't tried	Dislike at present
Tofu	☐	☐	☐	☐
TVP mince	☐	☐	☐	☐
Fromage frais, natural	☐	☐	☐	☐
Natural low-fat Bio yogurt	☐	☐	☐	☐
Natural whole-milk yogurt	☐	☐	☐	☐

This isn't intended to be a comprehensive list of all available 'healthy' foods, by the way, but it is a fair cross section.

Now look back through your ticks.

If you have some ticks in each list under the 'Like' or 'Will eat' headings, then you have a sound basis for forming a slimmer, healthier diet without doing much more. These are the foods that you can eat and enjoy without any problems and no more adjustments. Make the most of them!

If you have ticks under the 'Haven't tried' heading, well, great. Here is a marvellous opportunity for you to discover some new foods and make your slimming and weight maintenance diet more interesting. One of the keys to taking control of your diet and your figure successfully is the willingness to try some new things, and never to condemn anything until you have tried it. (See below for ways to incorporate new foods into your diet.)

If you have ticks under the 'Dislike at present' heading, don't be disheartened. Remember, you don't *have* to eat any of these foods (assuming you haven't ticked the 'dislike' box for absolutely everything!). By trying some of the ideas here you may find that, in fact, you can turn a 'dislike' food into a 'like' food.

*   *   *

> ### 'When I see available food, I eat it even if I'm not hungry.'
> ### 'Once I open a pack of something, I can't stop until it's empty.'
> ### 'I always eat up everything I'm given.'

If you often find yourself saying these things or feeling this way, you are an 'automatic eater', downing many unnecessary calories a day on 'automatic pilot'. Overcoming this habit alone may well be enough to help you lose weight with little need to cut the calories in other ways. And it's not difficult. Putting food into your mouth when you're not hungry – just thoughtless – is a habit. It may be a long-standing habit, but it is one you can control. Remember, food is an inanimate object with no mind of its own. *You* have a mind of your own. You can learn to say 'no'.

You can defeat old habits most easily by adopting this approach:

1. Learn to *focus* on what you are doing.
2. *Decide* whether what you are putting in your mouth is what you really want.
3. Say *'no'* to yourself (and others if necessary) by the easiest possible means available. Use 'props' or a 'step-by-step' approach if appropriate.

More of this 'focus-decide-say no' system in a minute, but first let's find out how often you eat on 'automatic pilot'.

Keep a record of everything you eat during the course of today or tomorrow. Write it down in the chart on the next page and fill out the 'reason' column. Leave the solution column blank for the time being.

To help you, overleaf is an example of how one mother might account for some of her 'automatic pilot eating' on a typical day.

We will return to your list at the end of the discussion and you can fill in your own solutions.

Food eaten	Time	Reason	Solution
Half a pack crunchy nut biscuits	9 a.m.	Opened pack for son's lunch-box. Ate without thinking	Will try to concentrate on what I'm doing in future
Fish portion in batter, fried	6.30 p.m.	Cooked it for child who said he wanted two and ate only one	Cook less in future – he often can't eat up all his food
Pack of mini choc eggs	8 p.m.	Fancied something sweet while watching TV. Didn't realise I'd eaten whole pack	Have a piece of fruit instead, or, put out 'allowed' amount of treat before I sit down

Your own diary

Food eaten	Time	Reason	Solution

Eating food because it's there

How many of these do you do? *Tick the statements that apply to you:*

☐ I take food that's offered me without even considering whether or not I want it (e.g., canapés at a drinks party – or, indeed, another drink at a drinks party)

☐ I keep dipping my hand into the peanuts or crisps at a bar or party or into the bag of sweets at home, until they are all gone

☐ I eat the roll and butter at a restaurant or the free mints afterwards

☐ I always eat a pudding after the main course because that is what I have always done

☐ I go to the café at lunchtime to buy a sandwich and I come out with a Danish pastry too, because the tray was right in front of my eyes

These are classic cases of 'automatic pilot' action, which we can defeat by returning to the three-step approach:

(1) Focus. (2) Decide. (3) Say 'no'.

Here are some examples of that system at work.

✱ **Beat** automatically accepting food that's offered.
   Focus on what you are doing. (I am about to accept food because it is being offered, literally, on a plate.)
   Decide. (Do I really need it? If I have a few of these, how will I feel? I only ate an hour or two ago. I'm going to say 'no'.)
   Say 'no' in the easiest possible way. (If a waiter is offering, it is no problem just to shake your head. If it's a friend, smile and say: 'I've just had one, thanks!')

✳ **Beat** the urge to dip your hand in the peanut tray (or whatever).

Focus on what you are doing. (This takes practice but learn to be aware of your hand moving to your mouth each time.)

Decide. (No, this is ridiculous, I've had enough of these nuts/crisps/sweets, so why am I eating them?)

Say 'no', using props (ask barman to take crisps away/move them down the bar yourself/get up and replace the taste with something else, e.g., a mint if you've been eating savouries). If the 'nibble food' is in the home, ask yourself: *Why is it in the home?* Have you been planning and shopping wisely?

✳ **Beat** the urge to eat all the extras during your restaurant meal. How easy it is to get through the bread basket while you decide what you are going to choose from the menu!

Focus. (I am getting through an awful lot of this bread and butter.)

Decide. (I am hungry but if I eat much of this it will spoil my appetite for the food I really want.)

Say 'no'. (Move basket to another table/ask waiter to take it away/get up and visit loo/take a drink of water.)

✳ **Beat** 'because I always have eaten desserts.'

Focus. (I'm eating this because I've been doing so for years.)

Decide. (I expect it's all these sweet things when I'm full that help to make me fat. I'd like to try to cut them down or out somehow.)

Say 'no'. (Perhaps use the step-by-step technique. First take smaller portions; then change to a lighter dessert – e.g., a yogurt – then to a piece of fresh fruit.)

✳ **Beat** the urge to buy extra when you go to the takeaway.

Focus. (I've come here for a sandwich but I can see those pretty pastries there. However, I know they have been put there just to tempt people like me.)

Decide. (I had no intention of buying one before I came in, so why should I change my mind?)

Say 'no'. (Use props to bolster your resolve. Find a different sandwich shop where they don't display the sweet foods under your nose. Or ask a colleague if (s)he'll buy your sandwich for you. Or take your own lunch to work.)

Cleaning the plate

Many people continue to eat long after they feel full up simply because there is still food on their plate. Other people will polish off leftovers on a similar principle, usually without consciously thinking about it. But I believe that for the young much of this attitude is an inherited one. The idea that it was a dreadful waste to leave anything on the plate began during the food-lean war years. Older readers may themselves remember those years.

Our next discussion about the difference between hunger and appetite will help solve this problem but you should also adopt the three-stage approach.

Focus: learn to concentrate on your eating and recognise the point at which you feel full rather than the point at which the plate is clean.

Decide: 'I have had enough to satisfy my hunger. If I have any more I will be eating unnecessary calories.'

Say 'no': stop eating. Remove the plate. Use props. If you prepared the food, obviously the answer is to put less on your plate. If you are a guest, ask the preparer to serve you a smaller portion. Should there habitually be a lot of food wastage in your house, you need to rethink at the planning and shopping stage and prepare a smaller amount of food for meals. Habitually buying and preparing too much food is a waste of money and resources – and eating it isn't the answer.

CHAPTER TWO

Say Goodbye to the Diet Mentality

Has Dieting (with a capital D) been an important part of your life up until now? Have you conducted a love/hate relationship with your food and an ongoing battle with your willpower over a Diet campaign – a battle that, sadly, has so far ended in failure?

Here you can learn to leave that thinking behind you for good and begin to develop a more balanced and more realistic approach to getting and staying slim.

It is important to understand that 'overcontrol' is just as bad as 'no control'. Overcontrol leads to a fight with food and, almost inevitably, to long-term failure. So here's where you learn to relax a little as you control not your diet but the wilder excesses of the hopes, expectations and resolutions that have been fuelled so long by the tyrannical diet industry. Here's where, once and for all, you rid yourself of the destructive diet mentality.

* * *

'I've already tried many diets – all fruit, liquids only, no food before noon, no protein with starch, etc. etc. and I've failed on all of them.'

Why do diets fail you? No, it isn't the case that you have failed on diets; the diets have failed you. They required you to be too tough on yourself and this prevented you from sticking to them.

Here are some of the reasons why these diets failed:

- You didn't like the foods they allowed.
- They didn't allow you the foods you like.
- You felt hungry too often.
- They didn't fit in with your lifestyle.
- They were ridiculous diets that, even if you followed them to the letter, wouldn't have worked anyway.
- They hadn't programmed you into a way of eating you could stick with – so any lost weight soon came back.
- After failing several times to help you lose weight, they made you feel you were programmed for failure.

The only way in which you 'failed' was in picking the diets in the first place, but, as you're not a nutritionist or health expert, how were you to know?

Also, have you succumbed to the power of the 'diet aid' ad? Have you tried mail-order slimming pills or any of the other 'cures' that promise weight loss without dieting such as slimming patches, sauna suits, special detoxifying potions, ear clips to stop hunger pangs, cassette tapes for slimming while you sleep, 'negative calorie' foods? Did you fail to lose weight on those as well?

'Diet aids' that promise weight loss without calorie reduction are not being honest and diets that don't fit in with you won't work. So stop blaming yourself and feeling inadequate. You can lose weight and you can keep it off just as well as anyone else can. All you need do is promise yourself that you will never try such a 'Diet' or 'diet aid' again.

Improving your outlook

To achieve the right frame of mind about slimming you need to recognise three things:

1. Weight loss does involve change – in the number of calories you eat; and/or the amount of exercise you take; and/or in the type of food you eat.

2. These changes need not be drastic and certainly need not be unpleasant.

3. For many people, changes in habits take time.

Don't think of losing weight as being on a diet. To slim successfully you must never, ever, wake up one morning (often a Monday morning, for some reason) and say: 'Oh help, day one of my diet!'

Yes, there are some people who decide they need to lose weight, embark on a diet, lose the weight and then get on with their lives. If you were one of those people, you wouldn't be reading this book. In your case there is *no* need to feel obliged to lose any set amount of weight during any particular timespan.

To overcome the diet mentality you need to:

- Start gently so you don't wake up one morning with that sinking feeling common to dieters of a tyrannical diet.
- Control your slimming campaign your way and don't take any notice of what other dieters you know are doing.
- Limit the fat content of your diet so that you can still eat plenty while you slim. Eating plenty is one of the keys to permanent weight control. The latest UK study as I write shows that people who diet on as much as 1,600 calories a day show better overall weight-loss results than people who try to keep to nearer 1,000 calories a day. This is because the people on 1,000 calories a day find it harder to stick to their diets (not because, as is often argued, low-calorie diets make you fat!).

  As long as your overall food intake is less – even if just a little less – than your energy output, you will lose weight. So in theory if you stay fat on, say, 2,250 calories a day, cutting down to 2,000 a day will still have you losing in the long run.

- Set yourself a reasonable goal weight. If you have a lot to lose, this should be towards the higher end of the height/weight charts and it will also help if you divide the total amount of weight you need to lose into 'manageable bits' and 'mini-goals' (say, a stone (6.4 kg) or even half a stone (3.2 kg) at a time).

- Aim to reach your goal (or mini-goal) in no specific timespan. It isn't *necessary* to get there in any particular length of time; you just need to get there eventually. This way you will avoid setting yourself unreasonable weekly weight-loss targets. It is very easy to say: 'I will lose 3 lbs (1.4 kg) a week' and then, if one week you only lose 1 lb (¹/₂ kg), instead of feeling pleased at the 1 lb (¹/₂ kg) weight loss you feel you have failed. As this point the likelihood of you giving up is greater.

So if you do prefer to set a weight-loss target, it is better to choose a low one and to consider your weight loss over a period of a month rather than on a weekly basis. This is particularly useful for women who have menstrual cycles as weekly weight readings can give a very false picture both because of pre-menstrual fluid retention and because of many women's natural need to eat more in the week or so preceding the period.

*   *   *

'I'm either very good or very bad when I'm dieting. I can be strict with myself for days, but then the willpower evaporates and I binge.'

How can you beat the all-or-nothing syndrome? Alternating periods of bingeing and virtually starving are typical of an obsessive dieting behaviour pattern. Many women do this (the pattern differs from bulimia in that sufferers don't make themselves vomit). It usually isn't an 'eating disorder' as such, it is simply your body telling you that it needs more food. You don't *need* willpower if you're slimming correctly.

The low-carbohydrate, high-protein diets of the 1970s first caused the binge/starve effect to become apparent and many women have since been alternately crash-dieting and bingeing.

The fact is that if you starve your body of carbohydrate foods for any length of time, you will inevitably end up with a strong desire to eat the foods you've been avoiding. This is in part due to the fact that a low-complex-carbohydrate diet (low on foods such as bread and potatoes) can lead to a relatively rapid reduction in blood-sugar after a meal – a condition that makes us physically desire a carbohydrate food to restore the balance – and what will restore the balance most quickly is a 'simple carbohydrate', a sugary food such as chocolate, sweets or biscuits. This dose of sugar will send the blood levels soaring quickly.

Also, of course, it is well known that when people are deprived of something, psychologically they want it even more. Doctors have likened people on strict diets to tightly wound springs: the harder they try to stick to a diet, the tighter the spring is wound and the more pronounced the breakdown of the diet when that spring is released. So you see, this isn't you being 'good' or 'bad', it is simply you reacting in a normal way to an overly restrictive eating pattern.

Very low-calorie, low-carbohydrate diets are in fact the very worst thing you can go on for long-term weight control and one of the quickest ways to mess up your body's natural balance. Promise yourself you'll never again go on any diet that severely limits your intake of complex carbohydrates (bread, potatoes, pasta, cereals, rice and pulses) or that asks you to eat less than three times a day.

Here are the guidelines for avoiding the binge/starve trap in the future:

- Aim for slow weight loss.
- Eat plenty.

- Eat regularly.
- Don't think of any food as 'forbidden'; just remember to restrict some foods (the high-fat ones discussed in section 1) to sensible amounts.
- Always eat something nutritious when you feel hungry.
- Remember there are certain times when you may feel hungrier than usual. If it is real hunger, don't feel guilty, eat.

PMS may make you feel hungrier than usual, and if your hungry patches regularly occur after your mid-cycle and disappear soon after menstruation begins, this is almost definitely the cause. Allow for it in your slimming campaign.

*   *   *

'I find diets so boring that even if I start off with enthusiasm I tail off after a few days.'

'Dieting makes me depressed and miserable, so it's no wonder I don't stick at it.'

I am always amazed at the number of people who are convinced that to lose weight they need to eat certain types of 'boring diet food' – things like cottage cheese, lettuce, celery, grapefruit, bran and crispbreads – and to drink only lemon juice and mineral water.

Now, personally, I like all those things (except for the bran!) from time to time as a small part of my diet, but I can quite see that if that is your idea of a diet you will be bored. You may very well be miserable too.

Neither does losing weight have to entail living on the same one type of food – say a glass of milkshake – for weeks on end.

And yet the person with the 'Diet' mentality will hardly believe that you can actually lose weight without eating like that. But that old idea that you must suffer misery and deprivation to attain a nice new figure is something to banish from your mind straight away. It's not true and this book proves it.

You will find your local library and bookshop well stocked with recipe books containing new-style, reduced-fat recipes to try.

Give it a go! Forget the old image of a 'dieter'. You are a person who wishes to lose some weight and you are doing so. Losing weight is nothing more than weight *control* applied a little more strongly. It isn't a secret land where only the fittest survive. Neither are you locked into a routine you hate. You can lose weight on the foods you enjoy best there are plenty you enjoy that are also foods you can slim on.

Slimming isn't a prison or a desert island. It is you exercising control in the way that suits you best. And knowing *why* you have overeaten is the key to knowing what does suit you best.

CHAPTER THREE

Eat to Slim

YOUR BODY PROFILE

The first thing we need to do is work out your body profile so we can gauge your Optimum Eating Level. Complete the chart opposite, then add up your score.

Now use your score to reckon your body type:

Score between 12 and 15: You are Type 1
Type one means that you are likely to have a very high metabolic rate and you should be able to eat more than the average person who wants to slim and still lose weight well.

Score between 8 and 11: You are Type 2
Type two means that you are likely to have a high metabolic rate and you should be able to eat a little more than the average person and still lose weight well.

Score between 4 and 7: You are Type 3
Type three means that you are likely to have an average metabolic rate. You will be able to eat well while you slim and lose weight at a reasonable speed.

Score between 1 and 3: You are Type 4
Type four means that you are likely to have a slower-than-average metabolic rate. The Eat to Slim plan will help you to lose

Sex   *Score*

Male: score 3
Female: score 1   ....

Age

Under 25:   score 3
26–35:   score 2
36–45:   score 1
46+:   score 0   ....

*Approximate amount of weight
you want to lose*

  5 st (31.8 kg) plus: score 4
3-5 st (19.1-31.8 kg):   score 3
2-3 st (12.7-19.1 kg) :   score 2
1-2 st (6.4-12.7 kg):   score 1
under 1 st (6.4 kg) :   score 0
(If you need help on this question,
turn back to pages 134–135)   ....

Height

6 ft (1.82 m) plus: score 5
5 ft 9 ins – 6 ft (1.75-1.82 m):   score 4
5 ft 6 ins – 5 ft 9 ins (1.67-1.75 m):   score 3
5 ft 3 ins – 5 ft 6 ins (1.60-1.67 m):   score 2
under 5 ft 3 ins (1.60 m):   score 0   ....

My total score is   _____

weight but you should aim for a slow to steady weight loss and
it is particularly important that you build more activity into your
life.

My type is ....

Your body type is important because it determines both your
likely weight-loss pattern and how much you will choose to eat
on the Eat to Slim plan. If you are very overweight your metabolic rate is likely to be high, but your age, sex and height all

have an important bearing, too. Put simply, the higher your metabolic rate, the more you should be eating on your slimming plan.

Many people who are very overweight find it hard to accept that they have a raised metabolic rate ('If I have a fast metabolic rate, why did I put on weight in the first place?'). But if those people were once slim (and all the other metabolism-boosting factors were average) their metabolic rate wouldn't have been particularly high. It is being heavy that causes the rate to rise. As you slim down, your metabolic rate adjusts and slows down too.

The reason the very overweight person should eat *more* on a diet is explained simply. Let's take an example. If you are, say, 4 stone (25.4 kg) overweight at 14 stone (88.9 kg), you have probably been eating up to 3,000 calories a day to maintain that body weight; by contrast, a slim person would maintain an average daily intake of about 2,000 calories. In scientific terms (and although bodies don't always behave exactly like this in practical terms, it is still a good guide), to lose 1 lb (0.5 kg) of body fat you have to create a 3,500-calorie 'deficit'; so if you took no extra exercise but simply ate 2,000 calories a day instead of 3,000, you would be creating a daily deficit of 1,000 calories or a weekly deficit of 7,000 calories, which equals 2 lbs (1 kg) of weight lost!

Therefore, a person weighing 14 stone (88.9 kg) at the start of the slimming plan could lose weight at the rate of 2 lbs (1 kg) a week while eating plenty. But if you were to do what many diets tell you and start on 1,000 calories a day, yes, you'd create a much bigger deficit and lose more weight, but by dropping your calorie intake to only a third of what you have been eating you would of course notice the big difference (even if you began eating the pyramid way), and you would feel hungry and probably not stick to the plan.

As your weight reduces, though, you do need to consume fewer calories a day as you approach your target. That is because, as we have seen, your metabolic rate when you were very big was artificially high, but as you get nearer normal body weight the metabolic rate also reduces in accordance with your new size. This means that in order to create that 'deficit' and continue to lose weight, you need gradually to reduce your calorie intake.

By this time, you will have steadily become accustomed to an intake of fewer calories and also to the adjustments in the type of food you eat, so it won't be a problem.

Activity levels also have a bearing on your prospective weight loss, so if you step up your energy output by becoming more active you will lose weight more quickly.

And one last point I need to mention about weight loss is that in the first week or two of any slimming plan you can expect to lose a lot more weight than in subsequent weeks. That is because in the first week or two the weight loss consists partly of fat but also of a lot of water, and glycogen (stored carbohydrate), which disappear as a natural reaction to reducing the calorie intake. The glycogen balance stabilises after a week or two, but if you are very overweight it could mean that in the first week of even a reasonably high-calorie diet you lose half a stone (3.2 kg) or more. Even people with only a stone (6.4 kg) or so to lose will experience a 3-4 lb (1.36-1.82 kg) loss in the first week.

So don't think after a couple of weeks that because your weight loss is slowing down you are 'failing again'. You aren't. You are now losing almost nothing but fat, which is what you want to lose!

THE EAT TO SLIM TRIANGLE SYSTEM

We have established that the higher your estimated metabolic rate, the more you need to eat to slim, and with this in mind I have devised a simple system of meals and snacks, all coded with triangles, so that whichever body type you are – 1, 2, 3 or 4 – you can pick a plan to suit yourself.

Each triangle represents 50 calories, and for each body type there is a wide variation in the number of triangles you can have in any day, depending on what kind of day you want.

These are the four grades of day to choose from:

Optimum, Steady, Easy and **Relaxed**.

Optimum   An Optimum day is one that I consider will give you your best weight loss, being realistic. The number of triangles I suggest you eat on an Optimum day is the minimum amount I'd recommend you to eat on any day while you are slimming.

If you try to go any lower you won't be putting into practice all you learned in Step Three. *Never* slim with fewer triangles than your Optimum level!

If you choose the Optimum grade *every day* of your slimming campaign you will achieve the *maximum* weekly or monthly weight loss that I believe is suitable for you.

Steady   On a Steady day you will be eating more than on an Optimum day, but you will still be creating a good calorie deficit and will still lose weight – albeit more slowly – even if you decide to choose Steady days throughout your slimming campaign.

Easy   An Easy day is one on which you will be eating more than on a Steady day, but will still be creating a small calorie deficit and will still achieve a weight loss that can be measured in terms of pounds over a month, even if you choose Easy days throughout your slimming campaign.

Relaxed   On a Relaxed day you will be eating more than on any of the other types of day. You will probably be eating about the right amount to maintain your current body weight – i.e., you won't lose any weight if you choose a Relaxed day, but you won't gain any, either!

So all you need to do to continue losing weight on the Eat to Slim plan is choose more Optimum, Steady or Easy days than you do Relaxed days.

Here is the triangle guide for each body type:

	Triangles per day			
Body type	OPTIMUM	STEADY	EASY	RELAXED
1	30	35	40	50
2	25	30	35	45
3	22	27	32	40
4	20	25	30	35

Choosing your days

Remember, this is the slimming plan that YOU use to suit yourself. You suit your day's slimming grade to what is going on in your life and how you feel.

It is best to decide beforehand which grade you will adopt for the following day, but the system can also work beautifully to take away the guilt on days when you ate more than you intended – something that happens to everyone, no matter what size or weight. If you indulge too much, you can simply count that day as a Relaxed day and carry on with the plan. Remember that as long as you have fewer Relaxed days than other kinds of day over the course of a week or month, you will lose weight.

Obviously, the more Optimum days you have and the fewer Relaxed days you have, the quicker you will lose weight.

It's totally up to you how you combine the days. For example, you could choose nothing but Optimum days and Relaxed days. Or you could choose mostly Steady days and a few Easy days but no Optimum and no Relaxed. You could choose all Steady; or perhaps mostly Optimum but some Easy.

I suggest that you choose:

OPTIMUM days when you are feeling strong, positive and happy and the day is fairly ordinary; also, where women are concerned, in the early days of the menstrual cycle.

STEADY days for as much of the rest of the time as you can.

EASY days when, if you're a woman, you're heading towards the end of the monthly cycle; or when you know that, because of, say, business arrangements, it isn't going to be possible to do an Optimum or Steady day.

RELAXED days when you just want a day off or it's a special occasion.

I prefer to think of a slimming campaign in terms of how you do over the course of a month, rather than how you do each week – particularly for women because of the vagaries of the monthly cycle. But that also is up to you. If you prefer to divide your days up on a weekly basis, then do so.

As you can see from all the triangle-rated meal suggestions in the pages that follow, you eat to suit yourself – big breakfast or small breakfast; large cold lunch or small hot lunch; main evening meal or light snack; several small snacks throughout the day and not one big meal at all .... The combination is up to you.

The only two *rules* that I'd like you to follow throughout your Eat to Slim campaign are:

- Always eat at least three times a day; preferably more.
- Aim to choose no more than 10 per cent of your daily triangles from the Red Extras list (see pages 67–72). That means, depending upon what Type you are and what grade of day you are on, you will be able to have from two to five triangles from this list.

Tips to help you

- Think about your 'hungry times of day' and plan your meals and snacks to fit in with them. Plan small snacks for times when you are least hungry.

- Don't be afraid if your body tells you it is hungry; if you feel the signs, then eat.

- If you plan to take exercise, don't eat a *big* meal immediately before, though a small-to-medium meal is allright.

- Begin the Eat to Slim plan gently. Start off with a few Relaxed days just getting into the swing of things. Then have a few Easy or Steady days before you begin on the Optimum days.

- The meal suggestions and recipes all follow, as nearly as possible, the 'new-style' pyramid philosophy, so you don't have to worry about that while you are eating to slim. The Red Extras give you your 'top of the pyramid' allowance of fat and simple sugars.

- Check through your store cupboard, fridge and freezer and run down your stocks 'old-fashioned-style' foods before beginning on the Eat to Slim plan.

- Buy only small amounts of the Red Extras so you can eat only small amounts!

- Try to plan ahead with your menus.

- Don't eat the Red Extras when you are hungry unless they form part of a bigger meal. Save them for after a meal.

- All the meal suggestions and recipes are based on my 'swops' principle, always using a lower-fat or lower-calorie food when it will do just as well as a higher one.

- If there is a food or snack you wish to include in your slimming campaign but it is not listed among the suggestions (see pages 47–75), then find out its calorie content (most commercial foods have a calorie value listed on the packet), count one triangle for every 50 calories and add it to the Red Extras list. If there is no calorie count given, look in at calorie guide, available in newsagents, or in the library. Or you could write to me, c/o my publishers, enclosing a SAE, and I will do my best to help you.

- I have tried as far as possible to provide meals that don't require much weighing of food, but you will need to weigh items from some of the meal selections – so check that you have a set of kitchen scales that mark ¼ oz (5 g) gradations. A set of measuring spoons is also a good idea, as is a measuring cup, since it's a much quicker method of gauging amounts.

- For those occasions when you eat out, there is a whole section of starters, main courses and desserts for you to choose from. Bear in mind, though, that the triangle guides are only approximate and that it is harder to stick to the pyramid method when you eat out. So class an 'eating out' day as a Relaxed day for the purposes of your slimming plan, even if you feel you didn't eat much!

- You may find it easier to stay with Optimum and Steady days if you plan plenty of meals and snacks based on the 'slow release' foods that take longest to be absorbed into your system. For instance, pasta, oats, most fruit, pulses, skimmed milk and yogurt are all 'slow release' foods, while other 'good for you' foods such as bread and potatoes are absorbed more quickly and may not keep you feeling so full up for so long.

- When choosing your daily menus, go for as much variety as possible so that you will get all the vitamins and minerals you need for good health.

- You can add Extras and Snacks to your main meals to make them bigger – e.g., add a soup snack to your lunch; or a fruit snack to your breakfast.

- Red Extras can be 'saved up' over a period of a few days. This is useful if you prefer one big 'treat' every few days rather than a little every day, or if you have a special

occasion coming up and you know you'll want to feel free
to eat or drink extra. If you want to save up your Red Extras
in this way, keep a record in your notebook.

Long-term slimming

If you have a lot of weight to lose, you may find you want to
widen the scope of your eating, perhaps by devising your own
recipes, or by using foods mentioned on the following pages but
in different combinations. In that case, please turn to page 105
at the end of the meals and recipes for the 'freestyle plan'. But
you shouldn't move on to this until you have been on the basic
Eat to Slim plan for at least two months and have recorded a
successful weight loss.

Right! Now fill out the details at the top of the chart on pages
48–51, plan your first few days (remember, start gently with
Easy or Relaxed days) and begin eating to slim.

UNLIMITEDS

Use these foods and condiments in unlimited quantities while
you are slimming and after.

Drinks   Black tea or black coffee (or with milk from Extras
list); herbal tea; fruit tea (no added-sugar kind); water, mineral
water; calorie-free 'diet' squashes and carbonated drinks
(though try to keep these to a minimum).

Eats   Celery, endive, garlic, lettuce of all kinds, cress; pickled
onions, yeast extract (Marmite etc.).

Condiments   Chilli peppers, chilli sauce (e.g., Tabasco);
herbs, dried or fresh, all kinds; lemons and lemon juice, limes
and lime juice; mushroom ketchup; mustard; oyster sauce;
spices, dried or fresh, all kinds; soya sauce; vinegar, all kinds;
Worcester sauce, tomato purée.

EAT-TO-SLIM RECORD CHART – WEEKS ONE & TWO

My body type is: _____

My weight: at start _____   Day 8 _____   Day 15 _____

Day	Today's grade				
1		△△△△△	△△△△△	△△△△△	△△△△△	△△△△
2		△△△△△	△△△△△	△△△△△	△△△△△	△△△△
3		△△△△△	△△△△△	△△△△△	△△△△△	△△△△
4		△△△△△	△△△△△	△△△△△	△△△△△	△△△△
5		△△△△△	△△△△△	△△△△△	△△△△△	△△△△
6		△△△△△	△△△△△	△△△△△	△△△△△	△△△△
7		△△△△△	△△△△△	△△△△△	△△△△△	△△△△
8		△△△△△	△△△△△	△△△△△	△△△△△	△△△△
9		△△△△△	△△△△△	△△△△△	△△△△△	△△△△
10		△△△△△	△△△△△	△△△△△	△△△△△	△△△△
11		△△△△△	△△△△△	△△△△△	△△△△△	△△△△
12		△△△△△	△△△△△	△△△△△	△△△△△	△△△△
13		△△△△△	△△△△△	△△△△△	△△△△△	△△△△
14		△△△△△	△△△△△	△△△△△	△△△△△	△△△△

1. Record your body type, the corresponding number of triangles for each grade of day (see page 43) and your starting weight at the top of the page.
2. Decide which grade of day you will aim for each day and write its symbol (0, S, E or R) in the left-hand column.
3. Cross off or fill in each blank triangle as you use it. Use a red pen for 'Red Extra' triangles. (50 blank triangles are illustrated but your chosen day may allow less than that, in which case ignore the 'spares'.)

My triangles allowed are:

Optimum ☐ Steady ☐ Easy ☐ Relaxed ☐

*Fill in the triangles as you eat to keep
a check of your day's total*

Grade
achieved

△△△△ △△△△△ △△△△△ △△△△△ △△△△△

△△△△ △△△△△ △△△△△ △△△△△ △△△△△

△△△△ △△△△△ △△△△△ △△△△△ △△△△△

△△△△ △△△△△ △△△△△ △△△△△ △△△△△

△△△△ △△△△△ △△△△△ △△△△△ △△△△△

△△△△ △△△△△ △△△△△ △△△△△ △△△△△

△△△△ △△△△△ △△△△△ △△△△△ △△△△△

△△△△ △△△△△ △△△△△ △△△△△ △△△△△

△△△△ △△△△△ △△△△△ △△△△△ △△△△△

△△△△ △△△△△ △△△△△ △△△△△ △△△△△

△△△△ △△△△△ △△△△△ △△△△△ △△△△△

△△△△ △△△△△ △△△△△ △△△△△ △△△△△

△△△△ △△△△△ △△△△△ △△△△△ △△△△△

△△△△ △△△△△ △△△△△ △△△△△ △△△△△

4. At the end of the day, record which grade you achieved in the right-hand column (which may or may not be the same as you had intended).
5. Weigh yourself no more than once a week – for women I suggest less often may be better.
6. At the end of the four weeks, record your new weight, add up the numbers of each kind of grade of day you achieved and compare the total with your weight loss. Use the information to go easier – or perhaps try a bit harder – next month, or to stay on the same track.

EAT-TO-SLIM RECORD CHART – WEEKS THREE & FOUR

My body type is: _____

My weight: Day 15 _____ Day 22 _____ Day 29 _____

Day	Today's grade					
15		△△△△△	△△△△△	△△△△△	△△△△△	△△△△
16		△△△△△	△△△△△	△△△△△	△△△△△	△△△△
17		△△△△△	△△△△△	△△△△△	△△△△△	△△△△
18		△△△△△	△△△△△	△△△△△	△△△△△	△△△△
19		△△△△△	△△△△△	△△△△△	△△△△△	△△△△
20		△△△△△	△△△△△	△△△△△	△△△△△	△△△△
21		△△△△△	△△△△△	△△△△△	△△△△△	△△△△
22		△△△△△	△△△△△	△△△△△	△△△△△	△△△△
23		△△△△△	△△△△△	△△△△△	△△△△△	△△△△
24		△△△△△	△△△△△	△△△△△	△△△△△	△△△△
25		△△△△△	△△△△△	△△△△△	△△△△△	△△△△
26		△△△△△	△△△△△	△△△△△	△△△△△	△△△△
27		△△△△△	△△△△△	△△△△△	△△△△△	△△△△
28		△△△△△	△△△△△	△△△△△	△△△△△	△△△△

1. Record your body type, the corresponding number of triangles for each grade of day (see page 43) and your starting weight at the top of the page.
2. Decide which grade of day you will aim for each day and write its symbol (0, S, E or R) in the left-hand column.
3. Cross off or fill in each blank triangle as you use it. Use a red pen for 'Red Extra' triangles. (50 blank triangles are illustrated but your chosen day may allow less than that, in which case ignore the 'spares'.)

This month I achieved:

Total Optimum days _____   Total Steady days _____

Total Easy days _____   Total Relaxed days _____

Total weight loss for month _____

Fill in the triangles as you eat to keep   Grade
a check of your day's total   *achieved*

△△△△△   △△△△△   △△△△△   △△△△△   △△△△△

△△△△△   △△△△△   △△△△△   △△△△△   △△△△△

△△△△△   △△△△△   △△△△△   △△△△△   △△△△△

△△△△△   △△△△△   △△△△△   △△△△△   △△△△△

△△△△△   △△△△△   △△△△△   △△△△△   △△△△△

△△△△△   △△△△△   △△△△△   △△△△△   △△△△△

△△△△△   △△△△△   △△△△△   △△△△△   △△△△△

△△△△△   △△△△△   △△△△△   △△△△△   △△△△△

△△△△△   △△△△△   △△△△△   △△△△△   △△△△△

△△△△△   △△△△△   △△△△△   △△△△△   △△△△△

△△△△△   △△△△△   △△△△△   △△△△△   △△△△△

△△△△△   △△△△△   △△△△△   △△△△△   △△△△△

△△△△△   △△△△△   △△△△△   △△△△△   △△△△△

△△△△△   △△△△△   △△△△△   △△△△△   △△△△△

4. At the end of the day, record which grade you achieved in the right-hand column (which may or may not be the same as you had intended).
5. Weigh yourself no more than once a week – for women I suggest less often may be better.
6. At the end of the four weeks, record your new weight, add up the numbers of each kind of grade of day you achieved and compare the total with your weight loss. Use the information to go easier – or perhaps try a bit harder – next month, or to stay on the same track.

Note: Artificial sweeteners such as saccharin and aspartame may be used if you feel they will help you (but try to limit these to avoid artificially prolonging a sweet tooth).

CONDIMENTS

Within some of the meal suggestions that follow, 'condiment of choice' is mentioned. In that case, choose what you like from this list. (They are each worth half a triangle and are already included in the meal triangle ratings.)
All 2 teaspoons only unless stated otherwise.

Apple sauce; brown sauce; gravy (from stock cube), up to 3 tablespoons; gravy (thick traditional), up to 1½ tablespoons; mango or other chutney; horseradish sauce; oil-free French or vinaigrette dressing, up to 3 tablespoons; low-calorie salad cream; mint sauce; sweet pickle; sweet and sour sauce from jar; satay marinade from jar; Slim for Life Light Mayonnaise (see recipe page 76); Kraft Thousand-Island-Style Fat-Free Choice; Kraft Thick and Creamy Mayonnaise-Style Fat-Free Choice; packet stuffing.

VEGETABLES

Within some of the meal suggestions that follow, 'vegetable(s) of choice' is mentioned. In that case, choose from this list. (They are worth half a triangle and are already included in the meal triangle rating.) *Unless otherwise stated, the vegetables should be raw, boiled, steamed, braised, microwaved, baked or grilled.*

Alfalfa sprouts; asparagus; aubergine; baby sweetcorn; bamboo shoots; beansprouts; beetroot; broad beans; broccoli; Brussels sprouts; cabbage of all kinds and Chinese leaves; calabrese; carrots; cauliflower; celeriac; chicory; courgettes; cucumber; fennel; globe artichokes; Jerusalem artichokes; French beans and whole green beans of any kind; kale; kohlrabi; leeks; mangetout; marrow; mixed frozen vegetables; mooli; mushrooms; okra; onions (including spring onions); peas, fresh or frozen; peppers, any colour; radish; runner beans; salsify; shallots; spinach; spring greens; squash; swede; tomatoes; turnips.

FRUIT ▲

All the fruit portions listed here are each worth a maximum of one triangle. Cross a triangle off your daily chart (pages 48–51) only if you choose a fruit as a separate item. When 'fruit choice' is mentioned within a meal or snack, its triangle value has already been taken into account within that meal.

Apple, 1 medium; apple, stewed using artificial sweetener, max. 140 g (5 oz); apricots, fresh or dried, max. 5; blackberries or blackcurrants, stewed using artificial sweetener, max. 140 g (5 oz); cherries, fresh, up to max. 110 g (4 oz); clementine, 1; damsons, stewed using artificial sweetener, max. 140 g (5 oz); dates, fresh or dried, 4; figs, fresh or dried, 2; gooseberries, dessert, raw, max. 75 g (3 oz); gooseberries, stewed using artificial sweetener, max. 250 g (9 oz); grapefruit, pink or yellow, half an average; grapes, max. 100 g (3½ oz); greengages, up to max. 5; kiwifruit, 1; mandarins or satsumas, max. 2; melon, one good slice or half a small; nectarine, 1; orange, 1; peach, fresh or dried, 1; pear, 1; pineapple, 2 rings fresh or canned in juice; pomegranate, 1; plums, fresh, max. 2 or stewed using artificial sweetener, max. 140 g (5 oz); raspberries, up to 200 g (9 oz); rhubarb, stewed using artificial sweetener, max. 175 g (6 oz); strawberries, max. 200 g (9 oz).

EXTRAS

Add these to your menu as you want.

▲

140 ml (¼ pint) skimmed milk
2 rye crispbreads
2 tablespoons diet coleslaw
125 ml (4½ fl oz, one average glass) unsweetened fruit juice

▲▲

275 ml (¹/₂ pint) skimmed milk
200 ml (7 fl oz) semi-skimmed milk
1 slice bread from a large medium-cut loaf with a little low-fat
spread
110 g (4 oz) potato, boiled, baked, or instant mashed
75 g (3 oz) [cooked weight] boiled rice or pasta equivalent to
25 g (1 oz) [dry weight]
(For Red Extras, see pages 67–72.)

SNACKS

Use these quick and easy snacks between meals or tack them on
to a Cold or Hot Meal to make it bigger.

▲

- 1 slice French toast or rye crispbread with a very little low-
  fat spread and reduced-sugar jam or marmalade
- 2 Crustinis
- 1 Sunblest Crisproll with Marmite
- 1 Hovis wholemeal mini-loaf with 1 teaspoon reduced-
  sugar jam
- 1 fruit from fruit list
- 1 diet fruit yogurt
- 1 diet fromage frais
- 100 g (3¹/₂ oz) very low-fat set yogurt with 1 teaspoon
  honey
- 1 rice cake topped with 25 g (1 oz) low-fat soft cheese and
  tomato slices
- 1 tub Boots Shapers Fresh-Fruit Salad
- Selection of crudités plus 1 Grissini stick dipped in 1
  tablespoon Kraft Fat-Free Choice Thousand-Island-style
  dressing
- 1 instant low-calorie soup plus 1 melba toast
- 1 can Weight Watchers minestrone soup

▲▲

- 150 g (5½ oz) natural low-fat or Bio yogurt plus 1 teaspoon honey
- Any two snack combinations from above list
- 1 Granose Apricot and Date Bar
- 1 crumpet with a little low-fat spread and reduced-sugar jam
- 1 small finger roll with a little low-fat spread and reduced-sugar jam or Marmite
- 25 g (1 oz) slice malt loaf with a little low-fat spread
- 1 large banana
- 1 mango
- 25 g (1 oz) sugar-free popcorn
- 1 Shape Twinpot yogurt
- 1 Weight Watchers soup plus 1 Crisproll

▲▲▲▲

- 1 average bap with a very little low-fat spread and 2 × 25 g (1 oz) slices extra-lean ham or with 2 low-fat cheese triangles
- 1 fruit teacake or bun with a little low-fat spread and reduced-sugar jam
- 1 large wholemeal pitta filled with chopped vegetables from list plus ½ × 113 g (4 oz) tub Shape Mexican-style cottage cheese
- 1 English muffin, toasted, plus reduced-sugar jam
- 1 pot ready-to-eat, low-fat rice pudding plus 1 medium banana
- 1 Boots Shapers Crispbread and Mushroom Pâté Lunch Pack plus 1 apple

BREAKFAST-TYPE MEALS

These vary from tiny breakfasts to big breakfasts. If you don't like to eat at breakfast time, perhaps you could have one at mid-morning instead (many are portable).

▲▲
- 1 diet fromage frais plus one fruit choice
- 1 diet yogurt plus 1 fruit choice
- 75 g (3 oz) natural low-fat yogurt with 25 g (1 oz) dried apricots or peaches or apples chopped in
- 1 Weetabix or 15 g (½ oz) puffed wheat with 100 ml (3½ fl oz) skimmed milk
- 25 g (1 oz) bran flakes or Fruit 'n' Fibre (using milk from Extras list)
- 1 slice wholemeal bread from a large medium-cut loaf with a little low-fat spread and reduced-sugar jam or marmalade or Marmite
- 1 large banana

▲▲▲
- Unlimited ripe tomatoes, halved and grilled, on 1 slice wholemeal toast from a medium-cut large loaf with a very little low-fat spread
- 1 large banana and diet fromage frais or diet yogurt
- Unlimited mushrooms, grilled or poached in a little vegetable stock and served on 1 slice toast as before
- 75 g (3 oz or 3 good tablespoons) natural low-fat yogurt with 1 portion fruit from list, chopped, plus 15 g (½ oz or average handful) muesli or Bran Buds
- 25 g (1 oz or average bowlful) unsweetened breakfast cereal of choice – e.g., corn flakes, bran flakes, Fruit 'n' Fibre – with 150 ml (5 ½ fl oz) skimmed milk or 100 ml (3½ fl oz) semi-skimmed milk
- 1 small banana, mashed with a pinch of cinnamon and a dash of lemon juice, on 1 slice wholemeal toast from a large medium-cut loaf (no spread necessary), warmed under the grill for a minute
- 1 slice bread or toast with a little low-fat spread and reduced-sugar jam or marmalade plus 1 fruit choice or 1 diet yogurt or fromage frais

- 1 portion (125 g [4¹/2 oz]) fruit compôte, made by
  simmering dried mixed fruit in water to cover plus 2
  tablespoons Bio yogurt and a sprinkling of bran flakes
- 140 g (5 oz) baked beans on 1 small slice wholemeal bread

▲▲▲▲▲▲

- 1 medium-cut, extra-trimmed back bacon rasher, grilled or
  dry-fried* until crisp; 1 × 75 g (3 oz) potato cake made by
  shaping instant mashed potato into a patty, dry-fried, *or*
  75 g (3 oz) baked beans; 50 g (2 oz) mushrooms, dry-fried,
  1 tomato, grilled *or* dry-fried; 1 wholemeal bap *or* 1¹/2 slices
  bread from a large medium-cut loaf with a very little low-
  fat spread
- 25 g (1 oz) muesli *or* 1 Shredded Wheat with 125 ml (4¹/2 fl
  oz) skimmed milk ; 1 slice wholemeal bread or toast from
  large medium-cut loaf with a little low-fat spread and
  reduced-sugar jam or marmalade; 1 portion from fruit
  choice *or* 140 ml (¹/4 pint) fruit juice
- 75 g (3 oz) smoked haddock fillet, poached or microwaved;
  1¹/2 slices bread from a large medium-cut loaf with a very
  little low-fat spread and 1 teaspoon reduced-sugar jam or
  marmalade; 1 portion fruit or 150 ml (¹/4 pint) fruit juice
- 75 g (3 oz) Greek yogurt topped with 1 teaspoon runny
  honey and 1 fruit choice, chopped; 1 average breakfast roll
  with a very little low-fat spread and reduced-sugar jam or
  marmalade
- ¹/2 grapefruit; 2 low-fat pork (or pork and beef) chipolatas,
  grilled; 100 g (3¹/2 oz) baked beans; 1 slice bread from large
  medium-cut loaf, plus a little low-fat spread

---

* *Dry-fried means fried in a non-stick frying pan which has been coated
with a very little oil (preferably corn or sunflower, or you can buy a cooking-
oil spray called Fry Light).*

COLD MEALS AND SNACKS

▲▲▲▲

- 75 g (3 oz) peeled prawns or tuna, chopped apple and 1 stick celery, chopped, all mixed with 1 level tablespoon mayonnaise dressing (see recipe for Light Mayonnaise on page 76, or use Kraft Fat-Free Choice), and green salad items of choice plus 1 medium slice bread
- Cheese and biscuits: 2 rye crispbreads, 1 cream cracker and 1 Crisproll with mixed salad of items from Vegetables list, plus *one* of the following: 25 g (1 oz) Brie, Edam, Port Salut or feta cheese; 2 reduced-fat cheese triangles; 25 g (1 oz) reduced-fat cheese of Cheddar, Danish Blue or Cheshire type; 40 g (1½ oz) Dairylea Light; 50 g (2 oz) Shape low-fat soft cheese (⅓ of pack); plus a little low-fat spread
- 75 g (3 oz) [cooked weight] cold pasta shapes mixed with chopped apple or 25 g (1 oz) small seedless grapes plus 50 g (2 oz) chunks tuna in brine, drained, 25 g (1 oz) red pepper, chopped small, all tossed in oil-free French dressing
- 1 Boots Shapers Tuna and Pasta Salad
- 1 Boots Shapers Tandoori Chicken Sandwich
- Salad sandwich: 2 medium slices bread spread very lightly with Shape low-fat soft cheese and filled with as many salad items from the Vegetables list as you like
- 1 average soft bread roll filled with 2 thin slices (50 g [2 oz]) very lean ham plus 2 tablespoons reduced-calorie coleslaw (see recipe for Light Coleslaw on page 76 or use commercial brand) and sliced tomato
- Roll filled with 25 g (1 oz) reduced-fat Cheddar-style cheese plus lettuce, chopped spring onion and 1 teaspoon sweet pickle
- 1 Boots Shapers Turkey Salad Roll
- 1 Boots Shapers Soft Cheese and Hickory Smoked Ham Bagel
- 3 rye crispbreads spread with 25 g (1 oz) Tartex pâté (any kind) and topped with items from the Vegetables list – e.g.,

sliced cucumber and radish; 1 fruit portion from the Fruit
list
- 1 half portion of Rice and Bean Salad (see recipe on page
80)

▲▲▲▲▲▲

- 1 whole pitta bread filled with 50 g (2 oz) hummus and
chopped raw vegetable items from the Vegetables list plus
side-salad garnish from Unlimiteds list
- Sandwich: 2 large (40 g, 1½ oz) slices bread with a little
low-fat spread and filled with items from the Vegetables list
plus 50 g (2 oz) lean cooked chicken or roast pork or ham
and 1 item from the Condiments list
- Salad bap: 1 large bap with a little low-fat spread and filled
with 25 g (1 oz) reduced-fat Cheddar- or Cheshire-style
cheese or 1 hard-boiled egg, size 3, and plenty of salad
items from the Vegetables list
- Sandwich: 2 slices bread from large medium-cut loaf filled
with 1 × 100 g (3½ oz) can tuna in brine, drained and
mashed, plus lettuce and cucumber; 1 fruit choice
- Bacon sandwich: 2 slices bread from a large medium-cut
loaf filled with 2 tablespoons Light Coleslaw (see recipe on
page 76) plus 1 slice back bacon, trimmed and well grilled
then crumbled; salad garnish
- Ploughman's: 75 g (3 oz) slice French bread plus 40 g
(1½ oz) reduced-fat Cheddar-style cheese or 1 whole 100 g
(3½ oz) pot onion and Cheddar cottage cheese; 1 teaspoon
pickle; tomato and celery
- 1 whole pitta bread filled with half a can of tuna in brine,
drained, plus 50 g (2 oz) red kidney beans or other beans of
your choice plus 2 teaspoons condiment of your choice (see
list) and chopped salad
- 25 g (1 oz) Italian Mozzarella cheese, thinly sliced and
arranged between 1 sliced tomato, topped with a drizzle of
oil-free French dressing and garnished with sliced black

olives and spring onions; plus 75 g (3 oz) slice French bread
- Takeaway: 1 Boots Shapers Back Bacon and Cream Cheese Bloomer, plus 1 apple; *or* 1 Boots Shapers Brie and Black Grape Sandwich, plus a fruit choice; *or* any chicken salad (no mayonnaise) *or* ham-and-tomato sandwich; *or* pastrami and tomato bagel; *or* Marks and Spencer Tandoori Chicken or Chicken Tikka pitta
- Salade Niçoise (see recipe on page 77) plus 1 slice bread from a medium-cut large loaf
- Hawaiian Rice Salad with Chicken or with vegetarian option (see recipe on page 78)

▲▲▲▲▲▲▲▲

- Triple-decker sandwich: 3 slices bread from a large medium-cut loaf lightly spread with low-fat spread and the first layer filled with 40 g (1½ oz) extra-lean ham and the second layer with 40 g (1½ oz) cooked chicken or 1 medium hard-boiled egg, both layers with lettuce, cress and tomato plus 1 condiment of your choice
- Ploughman's: 75 g (3 oz) French bread with a little low-fat spread; 40 g (1½ oz) reduced-fat Cheddar or Cheshire-style cheese or Brie; 2 teaspoons sweet pickle; 2 pickled onions; a large mixed salad of items from the Vegetables and Unlimiteds lists
- Sandwich: 2 large slices bread with a little low-fat spread, filled with 50 g (2 oz) cooked chicken mixed with 1 tablespoon Light Mayonnaise (see recipe on page 76) plus plenty of vegetable items; 1 fruit choice; 1 medium banana
- Salad platter: 200 g (7 oz) cold cooked new potatoes tossed in 1 tablespoon Light Mayonnaise (see recipe on page 76), *or* 125 g (4½ oz) cooked rice and chopped peppers tossed in oil-free French dressing; 50 g (2 oz, 2 average slices) lean roast beef or pork or very lean cooked ham; mixed salad of items from Vegetables list; condiment of your choice

- Pasta Salad with Crispy Bacon (see recipe on page 78)
- Rice and Bean Salad (see recipe on page 80)

▲▲▲▲▲▲▲▲▲▲

- Ploughman's: 100 g (3½ oz) piece French bread with a little low-fat spread; 50 g (2 oz) Brie or reduced-fat Cheddar *or* 25 g (1 oz) regular Cheddar or Stilton; 2 teaspoons sweet pickle; tomato, celery, onion rings and lettuce
- Salad platter: 225 g (8 oz) cold cooked new potatoes tossed in 1 tablespoon Light Mayonnaise (see recipe on page 76) or Kraft Mayonnaise-style Fat-Free Choice; salad of 50 g (2 oz) cold cooked sweetcorn mixed with 1 small chopped red pepper and oil-free French dressing; salad greens; 75 g (3 oz) very lean cold roast beef or pork or lean cooked ham *or* 100 g (3½ oz) cold cooked chicken (no skin) or turkey; plus 1 condiment of your choice (see list)
- 100 g (3½ oz) cold cooked chicken (no skin) chopped and mixed with 1½ tablespoons Light Mayonnaise (see recipe on page 76) or Kraft Mayonnaise-style Fat-Free Choice which has been blended with 1 teaspoon mild curry powder and 1 teaspoon mango chutney; green salad; 75 g (3 oz) French bread
- Prawn and Pasta Salad (see recipe on page 79)
- Rice and Bean Salad (see recipe on page 80) with 1 chopped hard-boiled egg added

HOT MEALS AND SNACKS

▲▲▲▲

- Any Weight Watchers canned soup plus 1 slice bread from a large medium-cut loaf; 1 fruit portion of choice
- 1 slice bread from a large medium-cut loaf toasted and spread with a little low-fat spread and topped with 1 medium poached egg *or* 140 g (5 oz, third of a can) baked beans *or* wholewheat spaghetti in tomato sauce

- 1 × 50 g (2 oz) beefburger, well grilled, in 1 average bap plus salad items from the Vegetables list and lettuce; 1 condiment of your choice (see list)
- 1 × 175 g (6 oz) baked potato split and topped with 1 good tablespoon 8% fat natural fromage frais and chopped chives
- 1 portion of Ratatouille (see recipe on page 81) with 1 average roll
- 1 slice bread from a large medium-cut loaf toasted and topped with 40 g (1½ oz) grated reduced-fat Cheddar-style cheese and sliced tomato and grilled until bubbling
- 1 can Campbell's Vegetable and Pasta Main Course soup; fruit portion of your choice
- 1 portion of Tangy Tomato Soup (see recipe on page 82) with 1 small roll
- Mulligatawny with beans: heat one 300 g (10½ oz) can Heinz oxtail soup with 1 level teaspoon mild curry powder and 50 g (2 oz) cooked beans of your choice (e.g., pinto, black-eye) or cooked brown lentils

▲▲▲▲▲▲

- 550 ml (1 pint) lentil and vegetable or lentil and tomato soup (e.g., New Covent Garden) plus 1 large (40 g [1½ oz]) slice bread
- 1 × 225 g (8 oz) baked potato filled with 140 g (5 oz) baked beans or chilli beans
- 1 × 225 g (8 oz) can Heinz barbecue beans on 1 large (40 g [1½ oz]) slice toast
- 175 g (6 oz) new or boiled or mashed potatoes; a large serving of any choice from the Vegetables list; 150 g (5½ oz) white fish of your choice simmered in a non-stick pan with a little white wine or a dash of wine vinegar mixed with 1 tablespoon water plus 1 firm tomato, chopped and 2 spring onions, chopped. Simmer until fish is tender
- Selection of vegetables of your choice from the list, cut into strips and stir-fried in a non-stick pan in 2 teaspoons oil, 1

condiment and spices of your choice, with 1 medium egg
added and stir-fried at last minute. Serve on 40 g (1½ oz)
[dry weight] egg thread noodles, soaked according to
instructions, or on the same weight of boiled rice

- 175 g (6 oz) mashed or baked potato with 1 medium serving
  of peas or sweetcorn or baked beans plus 1 portion of cod
  steak in parsley sauce or 150 g (5½ oz) any white fish
  baked in foil with herbs and lemon juice
- 1 × 100 g (4 oz) portion of New-Style Roast Potatoes (see
  recipe on page 82) with 2 portions of vegetables from the
  list and 1 small breast of chicken (no skin), baked
- Chicken Salsa Tacos (see recipe on page 83)
- Rice-Stuffed Baked Vegetables (see recipe on page 84)
- Italian-Style Roast Vegetables with accompaniment (see
  recipe on page 85)
- Indonesian Stir-Fry (see recipe on page 86)
- Chinese Beef and Red Pepper Stir-Fry (see recipe on page
  87)
- 50 g (2 oz) [dry weight] pasta of your choice boiled and
  topped with 1 portion of Tomato Sauce (see recipe on page
  88) plus 1 level tablespoon Parmesan cheese

▲▲▲▲▲▲▲▲▲

- 1 portion of Ratatouille (see recipe on page 81) mixed with
  65 g (2½ oz) [dry weight] pasta of your choice boiled and
  topped with 1 tablespoon grated Parmesan or 2 tablespoons
  Mozzarella cheese
- 1 × 100 g (3½ oz) gammon or bacon steak grilled and
  topped with 1 slice pineapple plus 75 g (3 oz) sweetcorn or
  peas, 175 g (6 oz) new potatoes and 1 condiment of your
  choice; 1 fruit choice
- 1 average beefburger, well grilled, in 1 burger bun plus 1
  condiment of your choice; 75 g (3 oz) oven chips; a large
  mixed salad of items from the Vegetables list plus
  Unlimiteds

- 1 × 175 g (6 oz) baked potato *or* 100 g (3½ oz) New-Style Roast Potatoes (see recipe on page 82); 1 medium chicken portion (no skin), baked (try using fresh rosemary and thyme with lemon juice to flavour); 1 portion of peas or sweetcorn; up to 2 portions of vegetables of your choice from the list; 1 condiment of your choice; 1 fruit choice
- Peppered lamb: 1 × 100 g (3½ oz) lamb steak with crushed peppercorns pressed into surface both sides, grilled; 225 g (8 oz) baked potato; either a large mixed salad or 2 portions of vegetables of your choice from the list
- 1 average pink trout fillet cooked in a non-stick pan in 1 teaspoon low-fat spread with 1 tablespoon chopped almonds added at last minute; 2 portions of vegetables of your choice from the list; 125 g (4½ oz) new or boiled potatoes
- 2 ready-made savoury pancakes (crêpes) filled with 1 portion of Chicken Salsa mixture (see recipe on page 83); a large mixed salad of items from the Vegetables and Unlimited lists
- Vegetable omelette: beat two medium eggs with seasoning and cook in a non-stick pan that you've coated with a brushing of oil, adding a variety of lightly cooked and chopped vegetables of your choice (e.g., courgettes, onion, leek) or raw salad vegetables (e.g., peppers, tomato, spring onion). Turn carefully halfway through cooking and serve flat with 1 large wholemeal roll or 50 g (2 oz) slice French bread and side salad
- Bean and bacon hotpot: grill well 1 lean slice back bacon and crumble it into a saucepan with 1 × 225 g (8 oz) can barbecued baked beans; heat and serve with 1 large wholemeal roll or 2 slices bread from a medium loaf
- Cauliflower and Bacon Gratin (see recipe on page 89) served with 40 g (1½ oz) hunk of bread
- Jambalaya (see recipe on page 90)
- Seafood Tagliatelle (see recipe on page 91)

- Spiced Pork with Rice (see recipe on page 92)
- Sweet and Sour Stir-Fry (see recipe on page 93)
- Seafood Crumble (see recipe on page 94) with 175 g (6 oz) new or instant mashed potatoes and green salad or green beans

▲▲▲▲▲▲▲▲▲▲

- 1 small ready-made pizza base topped with 1 portion of Tomato Sauce (see recipe on page 88) or half a ready-made jar of sauce, covered with 2 tablespoons grated Mozzarella cheese and a selection of sliced vegetables of your choice – e.g., mushroom, tomato, pepper, onion; serve with salad
- 4 ready-prepared barbecued spare ribs, baked or grilled and served with 50 g (2 oz) [dry weight] rice, boiled, plus 1 condiment of your choice and plenty of salad
- 1 × 225 g (8 oz) baked potato with 75 g (3 oz) lean roast beef or lamb or grilled steak or liver *or* 110 g (4 oz) lean roast pork or chicken; 2 portions of vegetables from the list; 1 condiment of your choice
- Beef and Vegetable Curry with Rice (see recipe on page 95)
- Vegetable Lasagne (see recipe on page 96)
- Pasta Spirals with Minced Beef and Vegetables (see recipe on page 97)
- Chilli Con Carne and Rice (see recipe on page 98)
- Chicken and Mushroom Risotto (see recipe on page 99)
- Pasta and Tuna Bake (see recipe on page 101)
- 3 low-fat pork chipolatas, grilled and served with 150 g (5½ oz) baked beans and 175 g (6 oz) instant mashed potato plus 1 condiment of your choice

▲▲▲▲▲▲▲▲▲▲▲▲

- Luxury Paella (see recipe on page 100)
- Double portion of any of the 6–▲ meals

DESERTS

▲

- 1 portion of fresh fruit from the list
- 1 individual diet fruit fromage frais (e.g., Boots Shapers)
- 1 individual diet fruit yogurt (e.g., Shape)
- 100 g (3½ oz) low-fat natural yogurt

▲▲

- 1 portion (up to 225 g, 8 oz) of fresh fruit salad with a squirt of aerosol cream
- 1 banana (cold or baked in foil with a little orange juice) plus a squirt of aerosol cream
- 50 ml (2 fl oz) ice-cream substitute (e.g., 'Too Good to be True') with 1 portion of fresh fruit from the list
- 1 Shape Twinpot
- Strawberry fool made by whipping 110 g (4 oz) fresh strawberries, hulled and chopped, with 100 g (3½ oz) natural fromage frais and a level teaspoon of fructose
- 1 Boots Shapers Raspberry Trifle
- 1 Boots Shapers Peach Sundae

▲▲▲

- 25 g (1 oz) dried apricots or peaches simmered in 50 ml (2 fl oz) water for 30 minutes then mashed including juices and served in the base of a wineglass topped with 2 tablespoons Greek yogurt and sprinkled with 1 tablespoon grapenuts
- 1 portion of Blackcurrant Cheesecake (see recipe on page 104)

▲▲▲▲

- 1 portion of Fruit-Filled Flan (see recipe on page 102)
- 1 Fruit Pancake with Creamy Sauce (see recipe on page 103)

RED EXTRAS

Biscuits

▲

1 fig-roll biscuit
1 Jaffa cake
1 chocolate chip cookie
2 Nice biscuits
1 gingernut biscuit
1 Bourbon biscuit

▲▲

1 Breakaway Milk biscuit
1 shortbread finger
1 Yo Yo biscuit
3 Rich Tea biscuits
3 cream crackers
1 Harvest Chewy or Crunchy bar

▲▲▲

1 Jordan's cereal bar
1 Penguin biscuit
1 Granose carob-coated fruit bar
1 Boots chocolate-coated cereal bar
2 Hobnob biscuits
2 digestive biscuits
1 Hobnob bar
2 chocolate digestive biscuits

▲▲▲▲

1 Chocolate Chip Tracker
1 Roast Nut Tracker

Chocolates and Sweets

▲

1 chocolate from assortment
1 toffee from assortment

▲▲

1 Lo Bar
1 fun-size Double-Decker
2 fingers Kit Kat
1 × 20 g (³/₄ oz) Cadbury's Dairy Milk bar
1 fun-size pack Maltesers
1 small bar soft nougat
1 tube Polo mints

▲▲▲

1 Cadbury's Fudge
2-bar Twix Teabreak
2 fun-size Wispas
35 g (1¹/₄ oz) bag Revels
1 tube fruit gums or pastilles

▲▲▲▲

1 standard Crunchie
1 Wispa
1 Cadbury's Cream Egg
1 Cadbury's Flake
1 tube Toffos
1 tube Smarties
1 Aero Chunky
1 standard (40 g, 1¹/₂ oz) bag Maltesers

▲▲▲▲▲

1 Cadbury's Caramel
1 standard Cadbury's Dairy Milk bar
1 standard Cadbury's bar Fruit and Nut
1 Lion bar

1 Picnic
1 tube Rolos

Desserts, Gâteaux, Ices

▲▲

- 1 × 125 g (4¹/₂ oz) French-style set yogurt
- 1 ice lolly
- 1 soft ice cream in cone
- 1 meringue nest filled with fresh fruit and a squirt of aerosol cream
- 1 × 150 g (5¹/₂ oz) pot Ambrosia low-fat custard or rice pudding
- 1 Bailey's Puddi
- 1 individual strawberry mousse
- 1 Boots Shapers fruit fool
- 1 × 100 ml (3¹/₂ oz) low-calorie ice cream or ice cream substitute plus 1 flat wafer

▲▲▲

- 1 Cadbury's Dairy Milk mousse
- 1 individual pot crème caramel
- 1 individual trifle
- 1 St Ivel Black Forest dessert
- 1 portion of Blackcurrant Cheesecake (see recipe on page 104)
- 1 × 150 g (5¹/₂ oz) tub Bio or fruit yogurt or Greek yogurt
- 1 × 100 g (3¹/₂ oz) tub fruit fromage frais

▲▲▲▲

- 1 × 100 g (3¹/₂ oz) slice Sara Lee Lite Cheesecake
- 1 × 100 g (3¹/₂ oz) slice single-crust apple pie with 2 tablespoons low-fat custard or Shape single cream
- 1 King Cone or Cornetto
- 1 Mars or Snickers ice cream
- 1 Thick and Creamy yogurt or Duet (twinpot) yogurt

▲▲▲▲▲
- 1 individual St Ivel cheesecake
- 1 × 75 g (3 oz) slice Black Forest gâteau or similar

Cakes and Bakery

▲▲
- 1 Mr Kipling French or Fruit Fancy

▲▲▲
- Bird's Eye Dairy Cream Eclair (frozen)
- 1 jam tart
- 1 small croissant
- 1 average slice carrot (passion) cake

▲▲▲▲
- 1 iced finger bun
- 1 average slice jam sponge
- 1 individual apple pie
- 1 average slice rich fruit cake

▲▲▲▲▲
- 1 jam doughnut
- 1 average slice chocolate cake

Alcohol and Drinks

▲
- 1 glass low-alcohol wine
- 1 average measure sherry
- 1 single measure spirits

▲▲
- 1 medium glass dry or medium wine
- 1 small glass sweet wine
- 275 ml (½ pint) beer or lager
- 275 ml (½ pint) cider

- 1 liqueur
- 1 can lemonade

▲▲▲

- 1 can coke

Sugar and Spreads

▲

- 2 heaped or 3 level teaspoons sugar
- 3 teaspoons honey or syrup or jam
- 2 teaspoons chocolate spread or peanut butter

Savouries

▲

- 1 heaped tablespoon grated Parmesan cheese
- 2 heaped tablespoons grated reduced-fat Cheddar or Mozzarella

▲▲

- 25 g (1 oz) full-fat cream cheese or Cheddar cheese or Stilton or Blue Brie
- 40 g (1½ oz) Edam or Brie or reduced-fat Cheddar

▲▲▲

- 1 packet crisps (25 or 28 g, 1 oz size)

▲▲▲▲

- 100 g (3½ oz) small portion average-cut chips

▲▲▲▲▲

- 1 samosa
- 1 spring roll

▲▲▲▲▲▲

- 1 standard-size Scotch egg
- 1 standard-size sausage roll

- 1 × 110 g (4 oz) slice quiche
- 1 buffet (party-size) pork pie

▲▲▲▲▲▲▲▲

- 1 average (150 g, 5½ oz) Cornish pasty

Fats and High-fat Items

▲

- 1 good tablespoon double cream
- 1 tablespoon reduced-calorie mayonnaise
- 15 g (½ oz) low-fat spread

▲▲

- 1 tablespoon full-fat mayonnaise
- 1 tablespoon French dressing
- 100 ml (3½ fl oz, average serving) custard
- 25 g (1 oz) low-fat spread
- 140 ml (¼ pint) full cream milk

▲▲▲

- 1 tablespoon oil, any kind
- 25 g (1 oz) creamed coconut
- 25 g (1 oz) taramasalata

▲▲▲▲

- 25 g (1 oz) butter
- 25 g (1 oz) margarine – any kind, including polyunsaturated, unless labelled 'low fat'

EATING OUT AND TAKEAWAYS

Starters

▲

- Fruit juice
- Plain melon

- Grapefruit
- Consommé

▲▲

- Vegetable soup – any kind except 'cream of'
- Marinated mushrooms
- Chinese-style soup (e.g., crab and sweetcorn)

▲▲▲▲

- French onion soup or minestrone
- Asparagus with butter
- Onion bhaji
- Samosa, small
- Stuffed mushrooms or tomatoes

▲▲▲▲▲▲

- Prawn cocktail (bread not included)
- Pâté and toast
- Avocado with prawns or vinaigrette
- 2 Chinese spare ribs
- Average Greek meze platter
- Taramasalata and pitta

Main Courses

▲▲▲▲▲▲

- Regular hamburger in bun from takeaway (no chips)
- Half a 10-inch (25 cm) pizza
- Grilled fish; new potatoes; green vegetables
- Grilled breast of chicken; new potatoes; salad

▲▲▲▲▲▲▲▲

- Individual pizza (5-inch, 12 cm deep or 7-inch, 18 cm crispy)
- McChicken sandwich
- Quarterpounder hamburger with bun
- Dolmades (stuffed vine leaves)

- Kebab and salad
- Mixed vegetable or prawn chop suey

▲▲▲▲▲▲▲▲▲▲

- 200 g (7 oz) steak or gammon steak, grilled (no visible fat); baked potato; salad (no mayonnaise)
- Chilli con carne and rice
- Carvery meal of lean meat and boiled potatoes with unlimited vegetables
- Scampi Provençal
- Salmon steak; new potatoes; peas; 1 tablespoon Hollandaise sauce
- Spaghetti Napolitana
- Calves liver; potatoes; green beans
- Cannelloni
- Chinese beef and peppers or chicken and beansprouts; half portion boiled rice

▲▲▲▲▲▲▲▲▲▲▲▲

- Chicken tikka with boiled rice
- Spaghetti Bolognese
- Spaghetti marinara
- Tagliatelle with vegetables
- Vegetable curry with half portion rice and 2 tablespoons dahl
- Ravioli
- Coq au vin
- Carvery roast including 2 chunks roast potato

Desserts
(Count these as Red Extras)

▲▲

- Fresh fruit salad or figs or lychees or mango
- Sorbet

▲▲▲

- Ice cream
- Meringue with fruit topping

▲▲▲▲

- Crème caramel
- Banana split
- Strawberries and cream

▲▲▲▲▲▲

- Fruit pie (single crust) or crumble
- Pavlova
- Chocolate mousse
- Trifle
- Lemon meringue pie
- Pancakes with maple syrup
- Gâteau

RECIPES

($\triangle$ = ¹/₂ triangle)

COLD DISHES

LIGHT MAYONNAISE

(Makes 8 level tablespoons at $\triangle$ per tablespoon)

50 ml (2 fl oz) natural low-fat yogurt
40 ml (1¹/₂ fl oz) reduced-calorie mayonnaise
2 tsp fresh lemon juice
1 level tsp dry mustard powder
Salt and black pepper

Blend all the ingredients together in a small bowl; store in a covered container in fridge. Will keep for a week or more.

Variations
- Add tomato purée for seafood dressing
- Add a little curry powder for Coronation Chicken dressing
- Add fresh herbs or garlic for stronger taste
- Low-fat Bio yogurt gives a creamier result in this dressing than most ordinary low-fat natural yogurts

LIGHT COLESLAW

(Makes 2 large servings of ▲$\triangle$ each)

110 g (4 oz) white cabbage, thinly sliced and chopped
1 medium carrot, grated
25 g (1 oz) onion *or* 2 large spring onions, finely chopped
15 g (¹/₂ oz) sultanas
3 level tbsp Light Mayonnaise (see recipe above)

Combine all the ingredients well in a bowl and store in a covered container in fridge. Will keep for a few days.

Variations
- Use 25 g (1 oz) chopped dried apricots instead of the sultanas
- Use red and white cabbage instead of all white

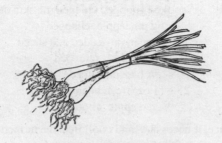

SALADE NIÇOISE

(Serves 2, ▲▲▲▲ per portion)

1 small head soft lettuce
200 g (7 oz) tinned tuna in brine, drained
50 g (2 oz) lightly cooked green beans
100 g (3½ oz) cooked potato
2 tomatoes
4 spring onions
25 g (1 oz) [good handful] watercress
4 tbsp oil-free French dressing
1 medium egg, hard-boiled and quartered
4 stoned black olives

Remove outer leaves of lettuce, then wash and tear them into pieces (discarding any that are poor). Cut the heart into four wedges and put all the lettuce into a salad bowl. Break up tuna and add to lettuce. Roughly chop the beans, potato, tomatoes, spring onions and watercress and add to bowl. Toss the salad in the oil-free dressing, then garnish with the egg and the olives.

HAWAIIAN RICE SALAD WITH CHICKEN
(Serves 2, ▲▲▲▲▲▲ per portion)

100 g (3½ oz) [dry weight] long-grain rice
or 275 g (10 oz) [cooked weight] long-grain rice
½ tsp ground turmeric
4 tbsp oil-free French dressing
100 g (3½ oz) cooked chopped chicken (no skin or bone)
1 ring pineapple, chopped
½ green pepper, de-seeded and sliced
1 stick celery, chopped
½ banana, sliced
25 g (1 oz) fresh beansprouts
½ red apple, chopped

Cook the rice, if necessary, and cool. Beat the turmeric into the dressing. Combine all the ingredients in a salad bowl.

Variation
● Vegetarians could use 100 g (3½ oz) [cooked weight] chick peas instead of the chicken

PASTA SALAD WITH CRISPY BACON
(Serves 2, ▲▲▲▲▲▲▲▲ per portion)

110 g (4 oz) [dry weight] pasta shapes of your choice
2 rashers lean-trimmed back bacon
½ red apple, chopped
1 small or ½ large ripe avocado, stoned, peeled and chopped
4 tbsp oil-free French dressing
20 g (¾ oz) ready-made croutons

Boil the pasta in plenty of salted water until tender (about 10 minutes). Grill the bacon rashers until crisp. Toss the apple and avocado in the dressing to prevent browning. Combine the pasta, apple, avocado and dressing in a salad bowl, crumble the bacon over and sprinkle the croutons on top.

PRAWN AND PASTA SALAD

(Serves 2, ▲▲▲▲▲▲▲▲▲▲▲▲ per portion)

150 g (5½ oz) [dry weight] pasta shapes of your choice
2 tbsp 1000 Island-style dressing (e.g., Kraft)
2 tbsp natural low-fat yogurt
Salt and pepper to taste
175 g (6 oz) peeled prawns
100 g (3½ oz) pineapple pieces
1 small green pepper, de-seeded and chopped
25 g (1 oz) flaked toasted almonds
Chopped parsley

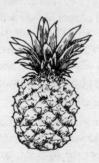

Cook the pasta in boiling salted water until tender (about 10 minutes), rinse under cold water and drain. Combine the dressing and yogurt with seasoning and any pineapple juice. Arrange the pasta, prawns, pineapple, pepper and almonds in salad bowl and toss with the dressing. Garnish with chopped parsley.

Variations

- Use melon chunks instead of the pineapple, in which case the calorie count will be a little lower
- Vegetarians could use 50 g (2 oz) Edam or 65 g (2½ oz) reduced-fat Cheddar instead of the prawns

RICE AND BEAN SALAD
(Serves 2, ▲▲▲▲▲▲▲▲ *per portion)*

This is good for using up leftover cooked rice and fridge odd-ments.

110 g (4 oz) [dry weight] brown rice
or 275 g (10 oz) [cooked weight] brown rice
100 g (3 ½ oz) [cooked weight] brown or green lentils*
4 tbsp oil-free French dressing
1 tsp curry powder
Chopped parsley or mint
Pinch caster sugar
50 g (2 oz) red kidney beans
1 small red pepper, de-seeded and chopped
50 g (2 oz) sultanas
50 g (2 oz) mushrooms, sliced
1 small orange, peeled and chopped
25 g (1 oz) cooked sweetcorn
Lettuce leaves

Cook the rice and lentils, if necessary; drain and cool. Combine the dressing, curry powder, herbs and sugar. Combine all the dry ingredients except the lettuce. Arrange the lettuce in the serving bowl and pile the rice salad into the centre.

Variations
● Use flageolet or cannellini beans instead of the kidney beans
● Use chopped dates instead of the sultanas
● Use white rice instead of brown, if preferred

* *To cook lentils or split peas: cover with water, bring to the boil and simmer for 30-50 minutes until tender. Drain and use as required.*

HOT DISHES

RATATOUILLE

(Serves 2, ▲▲ per portion)

2 tsp olive oil
1 medium onion, sliced
1 clove garlic, crushed
2 medium courgettes, sliced
1 small-to-medium aubergine, cubed
1 medium green pepper, de-seeded and chopped
4 tinned tomatoes and their juice
2 tsp chopped oregano
Salt and pepper

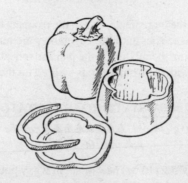

Heat the oil in a heavy-based, lidded saucepan or flameproof casserole and sauté the onion and garlic until soft, stirring frequently.

Add the rest of the ingredients and stir on a hot hob for a minute or two; then turn down the heat, cover, and simmer very gently for 1 hour. If the ratatouille looks dry towards the end of the cooking time, add some tomato juice or water.

TANGY TOMATO SOUP

(Serves 2, ▲▲ per portion)

400 g (14 oz) tinned chopped tomatoes
or 450 g (1 lb) fresh ripe tomatoes, skinned,
de-seeded and chopped
1 medium carrot, finely chopped
1 stick celery, finely chopped
1 medium onion, finely chopped
1 small red pepper, de-seeded and finely chopped (optional)
Dash of orange juice
Pinch of sugar
Pinch of ground coriander
Salt and pepper
50 ml (2 fl oz) passata
2 level tbsp fromage frais

Simmer all the ingredients, except the fromage frais, together in a covered saucepan until the vegetables are tender. Purée in a blender, return the mixture to the pan and reheat. Check seasoning. Serve with the fromage frais swirled on the top.

NEW-STYLE ROAST POTATOES

(Makes 400 g [14 oz], ▲▲▲▲▲▲▲▲ for the whole quantity,
▲▲ per 100 g [3½ oz])

375 g (13 oz) new or small waxy potatoes
2 tsp olive oil
1 tbsp lemon juice
1 tbsp chopped fresh thyme
1 tsp finely chopped garlic
Little coarse sea salt and coarsely ground black pepper

Preheat oven to 400°F/200°C/Gas mark 6.
  Scrub the potatoes, leaving the peel on. Cut them into small-ish pieces of about 25 g (1 oz) each, if necessary (if very small,

leave whole). Pat dry on kitchen paper and place in a roasting pan of suitable size (not too big).

Drizzle the oil and lemon juice over, then sprinkle with the thyme, garlic, salt and pepper, and, using your hands, make sure each potato is well coated with the oil and seasonings. If you can leave the potatoes to absorb the flavours for a while, so much the better.

Place in preheated oven and roast for 50 minutes, turning once, until golden and cooked through.

CHICKEN SALSA TACOS

(Serves 2, ▲▲▲▲▲▲ per portion)

175 g (6 oz) cooked chopped chicken (no skin)
25 g (1 oz) red kidney beans, chopped
2 medium ripe tomatoes, finely chopped
4 large spring onions, finely chopped
2 tsp corn oil
1 small green pepper, finely chopped
2 tsp lime juice
1 level tsp Mexican seasoning (or chilli powder) to taste
1 level tsp cornflour
1/2 tsp ground cumin
50 ml (2 fl oz) passata
4 taco shells
Fresh coriander or lettuce, chopped

Simmer all the ingredients, except the tacos and coriander/lettuce, in a small covered pan for 20-30 minutes. Heat the tacos in the oven; fill with mixture, garnish with coriander/lettuce and serve.

Variation
● The filling can also be used for pancakes, or over rice, pasta or baked potatoes

RICE-STUFFED BAKED VEGETABLES

(Serves 2, ▲▲▲▲▲▲ *per portion)*

75 g (3 oz) [dry weight] long-grain rice
or 200 g (7 oz) [ready-cooked weight] rice
2 medium aubergines
200 g (7 oz) chopped tomatoes with herbs
15 g (½ oz) chopped almonds or pine nuts
1 tbsp tomato purée
2 large spring onions, finely chopped
1 clove garlic, chopped
Salt and pepper
Passata and water (approx. 275 ml, 10 fl oz)
or tomato juice
100 g (3½ oz) tuna in brine, drained,
or pre-cooked brown lentils *or* 75 g (3 oz) lean chopped ham
1 level tbsp grated Parmesan cheese
1 tbsp chopped parsley

Cook the rice if necessary. Halve the aubergines and scoop out about half of the flesh. Chop and reserve this flesh. Add the aubergines halves to a large pan of boiling salted water and blanch for 3 minutes. Drain and pat dry.

In a saucepan, simmer the rice, aubergine flesh, tomatoes, almonds/pine nuts, tomato purée, onions, garlic, seasoning and a little passata for 10 minutes. Add the flaked tuna, lentils or ham. Place the aubergine halves in a shallow baking dish and fill with the rice mixture. Pour the passata mixed with water (or tomato juice) around the aubergines at the base of the dish. Cover with foil or a lid and bake at 400°F/200°C/Gas mark 6 for 1 hour or until aubergines are tender. Sprinkle the Parmesan and parsley over to serve.

Variations
● You could use large courgettes or de-seeded peppers instead of the aubergines and treat them in exactly the same way

- You can also use large tomatoes or mushrooms, but don't blanch tomatoes or mushrooms and be sure to reduce the cooking time

ITALIAN-STYLE ROAST VEGETABLES
with accompaniment
(Serves 2, ▲▲▲▲▲▲ per portion)

1 beef tomato, cut into 4 thick slices
4 large open-cup mushrooms
1 yellow pepper, de-seeded and quartered
1 small aubergine, cut into 2 cm slices
1 red onion, cut crossways into 4 slices
1 tbsp olive oil
Salt and pepper
1 clove garlic, chopped
75 g (3 oz) [dry weight] bulgar wheat
or brown rice *or* 50 g (2 oz) crusty bread
1 tbsp stoned black olives, chopped
1 tbsp sun-dried tomatoes, drained on kitchen paper
and chopped
Chopped thyme and parsley
4 tsp balsamic vinegar
1 tsp grated Parmesan cheese

Line a roasting pan with foil and place the prepared fresh vegetables on it. Put the olive oil into a saucer and, using a pastry brush, brush the oil over the vegetables. Sprinkle some salt, black pepper and garlic on the top. Roast for 20-30 minutes or until the vegetables are well browned and soft throughout. Meanwhile, soak the bulgar wheat or cook the rice and keep it warm. Serve the vegetables with the olives, sun-dried tomatoes, herbs, vinegar, any remaining olive oil, and Parmesan cheese sprinkled over, alongside the wheat or rice or bread.

Variations
- You can try other vegetables, such as globe artichokes or courgettes, cooked this way
- You can also try grilling them for a slightly different result, or, of course, barbecuing

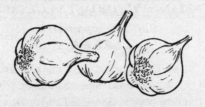

INDONESIAN STIR-FRY

(Serves 2, ▲▲▲▲▲▲ per portion)

65 g (2¹/₂ oz) [dry weight] fragrant rice
2 tsp corn oil
100 g (3¹/₂ oz) turkey or chicken (no skin),
cut into small strips
8 baby sweetcorns
1 carrot, cut into thin strips
100 g (3¹/₂ oz) fresh beansprouts
1 red pepper, de-seeded and finely chopped
50 g (2 oz) peeled prawns
4 spring onions, chopped
1 clove garlic, crushed
1 tbsp light soya sauce
1 tsp 7-Spice seasoning
Pinch of sugar
2 tbsp (or as necessary) chicken stock

Cook the rice in boiling salted water until tender; rinse in colander and set aside.

Heat the oil in a non-stick pan and stir-fry the poultry and sweetcorn until the meat is lightly golden. Add the rest of the ingredients and stir-fry for further 3 minutes. Add the drained rice and stir for 1 minute. Extra chicken stock can be added at any time if the mixture looks too dry or if it sticks.

CHINESE BEEF AND RED PEPPER STIR-FRY

(Serves 2, ▲▲▲▲▲▲ *per portion)*

65 g (2½ oz) [dry weight] egg thread noodles
2 tsp corn or sesame oil
125 g (4½ oz) lean beef steak, cut into strips
1 large red pepper, de-seeded and cut into large thick strips
6 spring onions, cut in half lengthways
50 g (2 oz) beansprouts
2 tbsp sweetcorn
1 tbsp oyster sauce
2 tsp light soya sauce
50 ml (2 fl oz) beef stock

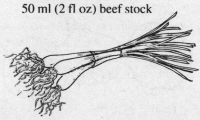

Soak the noodles according to the pack instructions (usually about 5 minutes).

Head the oil in a non-stick wok or frying pan and stir-fry the beef, red pepper and onion until the beef is brown (about 3 minutes). Add the rest of the ingredients, turn the heat down and stir-fry for 1 minute. Add the noodles to the pan, with a little more beef stock if necessary, stir and serve.

Variation
- You can serve the Beef Stir-Fry with boiled rice instead of noodles if you prefer. In that case, don't add the rice to the frying pan but serve it separately, precooked

TOMATO SAUCE

(Makes 4 servings of ▲△ each.
Freeze what you don't need)

1 tbsp olive oil
1 onion, finely chopped
Dash of white wine
400 g (14 oz) tinned chopped tomatoes
1 tsp Worcester sauce
1 clove garlic, crushed
1 tsp brown sugar
1 tbsp tomato purée
1 tsp chopped basil
Salt and black pepper

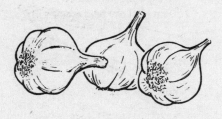

Heat the oil in a saucepan, add the onion and stir until soft. Add the rest of the ingredients and stir and simmer for 20 minutes until you have a rich sauce. Check seasoning. For a smoother result, press the sauce through a sieve.

Variations
- Add chopped and de-seeded red chilli for a hot sauce
- Add sliced black olives for a quick Italian pasta sauce

CAULIFLOWER AND BACON GRATIN
(Serves 2, ▲▲▲▲▲▲ per portion)

2 slices lean back bacon, trimmed of fat
1 small-to-medium (approx. 275 g [10 oz]
prepared weight) cauliflower, cut into florets
75 g (3 oz) whole green beans, cut into 2 cm (1 inch) pieces
1 quantity (2 portions) Cheese Sauce (see following recipe)
15 g (½ oz) reduced-fat Cheddar cheese, grated
25 g (1 oz) brown breadcrumbs

Grill the bacon until crisp, then crumble it. Boil or microwave
the cauliflower and beans until barely tender and arrange in two
gratin dishes with the bacon scattered over. Pour on top the
cheese sauce, scatter over the extra cheese and breadcrumbs
and grill until golden.

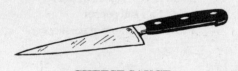

CHEESE SAUCE
(Serves 2, ▲▲▲ per portion)

15 g (½ oz) low-fat spread
15 g (½ oz) plain flour
175 ml (6 fl oz) skimmed milk at room temperature
30 g (1 ¼ oz) reduced-fat Cheddar cheese, grated
Salt and pepper to taste

Melt the low-fat spread in a saucepan, add the flour and cook,
stirring, for a minute. Slowly add the milk and stir until the con-
sistency is thick. Add the cheese and seasoning and stir until the
cheese melts. Check for seasoning.

This cheese sauce can be used in all kinds of savoury dishes
– e.g., over pancakes, with plain fish or to top moussaka and
lasagne.

JAMBALAYA
(Serves 2, ▲▲▲▲▲▲▲▲ *per portion)*

2 tsp corn oil
1 boneless chicken breast (approx. 110 g [4 oz]),
cut into small cubes
110 g (4 oz) pork fillet, cut into small cubes
1 small onion, very finely chopped
4 spring onions, chopped
1 stick celery, chopped
1 tsp Cajun seasoning
1 clove garlic, chopped
110 g (4 oz) [dry weight] long-grain rice,
boiled and drained
2 tomatoes, skinned and chopped
50 ml (2 fl oz) chicken stock
Salt and pepper
1 tbsp fresh chopped parsley

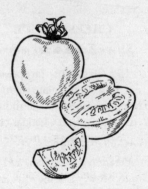

Heat the oil in a non-stick frying pan and fry the chicken, pork, onion and spring onion on a hot hob, stirring frequently. Turn the heat down and add the rest of the ingredients. Cook for 5 minutes, stirring frequently. Check for seasoning and serve.

SEAFOOD TAGLIATELLE

(Serves 2, ▲▲▲▲▲▲▲▲▲ *per portion)*

125 g (4 ½ oz) [dry weight] tagliatelle
2 tsp olive oil
1 small onion, very finely chopped
1 clove garlic, crushed
Pinch of saffron powder
2 tbsp dry white wine
50 g (2 oz) broccoli florets
25 g (1 oz) petit pois
50 g (2 oz) button mushrooms, sliced
80 g (3 ¼ oz) peeled prawns
4 crab sticks, thawed and chopped
25 g (1 oz) shelled mussels (thawed if frozen)
2 tsp lemon juice
2 tbsp skimmed milk
Salt and pepper
2 tbsp extra-thick single cream
or reduced-calorie double cream

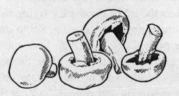

Cook the tagliatelle in boiling salted water for 10 minutes or until it is just soft. Drain in colander.

While the pasta is cooking, heat the oil in a non-stick frying pan and stir-fry the onion until soft. Add the garlic, saffron and wine and allow the mixture to bubble for a minute. Add the broccoli, peas and mushrooms and stir for 2 minutes. Add all the seafood, lemon juice and milk and simmer for 2-3 minutes until the fish is heated through. Add the seasoning and cream, stir, check the seasoning, and serve over the drained pasta.

SPICED PORK WITH RICE

(Serves 2, ▲▲▲▲▲▲▲▲▲ per portion)

125 g (4 ½ oz) [dry weight] ready-mixed
long-grain and wild rice
2 tsp corn oil
1 small red pepper, de-seeded
and finely chopped
1 small onion, finely chopped
140 g (5 oz) pork fillet, cubed
1 heaped tsp garam masala (or to taste)
110 g (4 oz) button mushrooms, halved
1 tsp French mustard
50 ml (2 fl oz) chicken stock
2 tsp lemon juice
Salt and pepper
2 heaped tbsp Greek yogurt or sour cream
Chopped fresh coriander or parsley

Boil the rice according to the packet instructions (usually about 20 minutes). Drain when wild rice is tender.

Meanwhile, heat the oil in a non-stick frying pan and fry the red pepper and onion until soft, stirring. Set to one side of the pan and add the pork. Cook over high heat, turning the pork cubes until they are brown on all sides. Turn the heat down, add the garam masala and stir. Add the mushrooms, mustard, stock, lemon juice and seasoning and simmer on Low for 5 minutes. When pork is tender, add yogurt or sour cream, stir and bring gently to simmer. Serve immediately over the rice, garnished with the coriander/parsley.

Variations
• You can use chicken fillet in this recipe, too
• Alternatively, try the basic recipe but use Hungarian paprika instead of the garam masala

SWEET AND SOUR STIR-FRY

(Serves 2, ▲▲▲▲▲▲▲▲ *per portion)*

110 g (4 oz) [dry weight] long-grain rice
or egg thread noodles
2 tsp corn oil
1 medium carrot, cut into matchsticks
1 small red pepper, de-seeded and sliced
50 g (2 oz) small broccoli florets
50 g (2 oz) baby sweetcorn cobs
50 g (2 oz) green beans, halved
50 g (2 oz) tinned bamboo shoots
4 spring onions, halved lengthways
3 Chinese leaves, sliced
75 g (3 oz) mushrooms, sliced
15 g (1/2 oz) flaked almonds

Sweet-and-Sour Sauce
1 rounded tsp cornflour
1 level tbsp runny honey
50 ml (2 fl oz) orange juice
1 tbsp light soya sauce
1 1/2 tbsp white-wine vinegar
1 tbsp white wine
2 tsp tomato purée

Mix all the sauce ingredients together in a bowl and set aside. If using rice, put it on the boil, or soak the noodles and set aside.

Heat the oil in a non-stick frying pan or wok. Stir-fry the carrot, red pepper, broccoli, sweetcorn and green beans for 3 minutes. Add the bamboo shoots, spring onions, Chinese leaves and mushrooms and stir again for 1 minute. Add the almonds and the sweet-and-sour sauce and stir for 1 minute or until sauce has thickened. If using noodles, add to the wok to reheat for a few seconds. If using rice, serve the sweet-and-sour vegetables over the rice.

Variation
- Use 100 g (3½ oz) firm white cubed fish instead of the almonds, or you could use firm tofu. In either case, add it to the pan with the first batch of vegetables

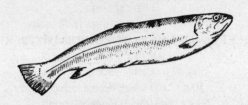

SEAFOOD CRUMBLE
(Serves 2, ▲▲▲▲▲▲ per portion)

100 g (3½ oz) broccoli florets
275 g (10 oz) cod or other white fish fillet
25 g (1 oz) peeled prawns
75 g (3 oz) button mushrooms, halved
4 spring onions, chopped
100 g (3½ oz) Greek yogurt
2 tbsp skimmed milk
2 tsp lemon juice
1 tsp cornflour
Salt and pepper
1 tbsp chopped parsley
1 tsp chopped dill
1 clove garlic, crushed
40 g (1½ oz) reduced-fat Cheddar cheese, grated
25 g (1 oz) brown breadcrumbs

Boil the broccoli until just soft, drain and reserve. Poach or microwave the fish until just cooked and flake it into 2 individual gratin dishes. Add the broccoli, prawns, raw mushrooms and onion to the dishes, dividing equally. In a bowl, mix together the yogurt, milk, lemon juice, cornflour, salt, pepper, parsley, dill, garlic and half the cheese until well combined. Pour the mixture over the fish and vegetables. Top with the breadcrumbs and remaining cheese and bake at 400°F/200°C/Gas mark 6 until the top is golden (about 20 minutes).

BEEF AND VEGETABLE CURRY WITH RICE

(Serves 2, ▲▲▲▲▲▲▲▲▲▲▲ *per portion)*

2 tsp corn oil
1 onion, chopped
175 g (6 oz) extra-lean braising beef, cubed
1 clove garlic, crushed
2 tsp curry powder (or to taste)
75 g (3 oz) potato, parboiled and cubed
100 g (3½ oz) cauliflower florets
or aubergine, cubed
50 g (2 oz) green beans
200 g (7 oz) tinned chopped tomatoes
1 tbsp tomato purée
40 g (1½ oz) [dry weight] brown, green or red lentils
or split peas
Pinch of brown sugar
110 ml (4 fl oz) beef stock
Salt
100 g (3½ oz) [dry weight] long-grain rice

Heat the oil in a non-stick pan and fry the onion until soft. Add the beef and fry till brown. Turn the heat down and add the garlic and curry powder; stir for 1 minute. Add the potato, cauliflower, beans, tomatoes, tomato purée, lentils, sugar and beef stock. Cover and simmer for 1 hour or until everything is tender. (Check after approx. 45 minutes that the curry isn't drying out; if it is, add a little water or beef stock.) Add salt to taste. Meanwhile, boil the rice and serve with the curry.

VEGETABLE LASAGNE

(Serves 2, ▲▲▲▲▲▲▲▲▲▲▲▲ per portion)

2 tsp olive oil
1 small onion, finely chopped
1 large courgette, sliced
1 small aubergine, sliced
1 small red or green pepper, de-seeded and chopped
75 g (3 oz) [dry weight] green or brown lentils
300 ml (11 fl oz) vegetable stock made with cube
200 g (7 oz) tinned chopped tomatoes
1 level tbsp tomato purée
1/2 tsp ground coriander
1 tsp oregano
Salt and pepper
4 sheets 'no-precook' lasagne
1 portion Cheese Sauce (see recipe on page 89)
2 tbsp Parmesan cheese

Heat the oil in a non-stick pan and stir-fry the onion until soft. Add the courgette, aubergine and pepper and stir-fry for 1 minute. Add the lentils, stock, tomatoes, tomato purée, herbs and seasoning. Stir, cover and simmer gently for 40-50 minutes until the vegetables and lentils are tender and the sauce is rich but quite runny (this is because the lasagne sheets absorb liquid). If the sauce is too thick, add a little water or stock. In 2 individual lasagne dishes (or a suitable shallow baking dish) put half the vegetable mixture in the base and cover each with a lasagne sheet. Cover with the remaining vegetable mix and remaining lasagne sheets, top with the cheese sauce to cover completely, then sprinkle the grated cheese over. Bake at 375°F/190°C/Gas mark 5 until the top is golden and bubbling (about 25 minutes).

Variation
● Try precooked haricot beans instead of the lentils – in which case, reduce the quantity of stock to approx. 200 ml (7 fl oz)

PASTA SPIRALS WITH MINCED BEEF
AND VEGETABLES
(Serves 2, ▲▲▲▲▲▲▲▲▲▲▲ per portion)

1 quantity (2 portions) Basic Minced Beef
(see following recipe)
200 g (7 oz) tinned chopped tomatoes
50 g (2 oz) sweetcorn *or* tinned borlotti beans, drained
25 g (1 oz) petit pois
50 g (2 oz) green beans, cut into 2 cm pieces
125 g (4½ oz) [dry weight] tricolour pasta spirals
2 tsp Parmesan cheese

Mix the minced beef with all the vegetables and simmer in a pan
for 10 minutes while you cook the pasta in boiling salted water.
Serve the beef and vegetables tossed with the spirals and sprinkled with the Parmesan cheese.

BASIC MINCED BEEF
(Serves 2, ▲▲▲▲ per portion)

Enough corn oil to brush on a non-stick frying pan
(or use Fry Light spray)
175 g (6 oz) extra-lean minced beef
1 medium onion, finely chopped
1 stick celery, finely chopped
1 small carrot, finely chopped
150 ml (5½ fl oz) beef stock made with cube
1 tbsp tomato purée
1 tsp Mediterranean herbs
1 tsp Worcester sauce
Salt and black pepper

Coat the non-stick pan with the oil and heat gently. Add the
mince and brown it over a medium heat, stirring from time to
time. Remove the mince with a slatted spoon when well

browned, leaving any fat which has run from the meat. In this fat, stir-fry the onion until soft (about 5 minutes). Add the celery and carrot and 1 tablespoon of the stock, and stir again for a few minutes. Return the mince to the pan and add the rest of the ingredients. Stir well and simmer for 20 minutes or until you have a rich minced beef sauce.

Variations
- This basic minced beef can be used for all kinds of dishes – e.g., cottage pie, or to fill a filo pie, or with the addition of some garlic and a dash of wine it makes a good Bolognese sauce
- Mixed with rice, it's a good stuffed vegetable filling, or try it in pancakes topped with Cheese Sauce (see recipe on page 99)

CHILLI CON CARNE AND RICE

(Serves 2, ▲▲▲▲▲▲▲▲▲▲▲ per portion)

1 large green pepper, de-seeded and chopped
150 g (5½ oz) [drained weight] tinned red kidney beans
200 g (7 oz) tinned chopped tomatoes
1 tsp chilli powder (or to taste),
or 1 whole fresh chilli, chopped
1 portion Basic Minced Beef (see preceding recipe)
110 g (4 oz) [dry weight] long-grain rice

Mix the green pepper, beans, tomato and chilli into the minced beef and simmer in a pan for 20 minutes while you cook the rice. Serve the chilli with the rice.

Variations
- Fresh chillis are widely available now and often have a better flavour than dried powder, but unless you like your chilli very hot, remove the seeds before chopping the chilli. You can also use dried whole chilies, for which the same applies

- TVP or VegeMince can be used instead of beef mince in all these recipes based on mince
- Try black-eye beans or borlotti beans in your chilli

CHICKEN AND MUSHROOM RISOTTO

(Serves 2, ▲▲▲▲▲▲▲▲▲▲ *per portion)*

1 tbsp olive oil *or* 15 g (¹/₂ oz)butter
1 smallish onion, finely chopped
110 g (4 oz) lean chicken fillet,
chopped into small cubes
175 g (6 oz) [dry weight] risotto rice
Dash of dry wine
500 ml (18 fl oz) chicken stock
25 g (1 oz) lean ham, cut into small strips
175 g (6 oz) mushrooms
(preferably at least two kinds),
sliced or torn
25 g (1 oz) petit pois
1 tsp chopped basil
A little salt to taste (optional)
Black pepper

Heat the oil in a non-stick frying pan and fry the onion until soft. Add the chicken and stir until tinged gold. Add the rice and stir for 1 minute. Add the wine and bring to bubbling. Add two-thirds of the stock, ham, mushrooms, peas, basil and seasoning, and stir the mixture; simmer gently, stirring from time to time. Add more stock as necessary. The risotto is cooked when most of the stock is absorbed and the rice is tender and creamy.

Variation
- Vegetarians can omit the chicken, use vegetable stock and top the risotto with 3 tablespoons of Parmesan cheese

LUXURY PAELLA

(Serves 2, ▲▲▲▲▲▲▲▲▲▲▲▲ *per portion)*

6 giant prawns
or 75 g (3 oz) peeled prawns
8 mussels, fresh in shells
or 12 frozen mussels, thawed
1½ tbsp olive oil
100 g (3½ oz) chicken or pork fillet,
cut into bite-sized cubes
1 small onion, chopped
1 small red pepper, de-seeded and chopped
Approx. 550 ml (1 pint) chicken or fish stock
1 clove garlic, crushed
1 sachet saffron
Pinch of paprika
150 g (5½ oz) [dry weight] long-grain rice
1 large tomato, chopped
25 g (1 oz) peas
100 g (3½ oz) firm white fish
(e.g., monkfish, swordfish or cod)
4 cooked or tinned artichoke hearts
1 tbsp chopped parsley
Salt and pepper

If peeling the prawns yourself, leave the tails on. If necessary, prepare the fresh mussels.

Heat the oil in a paella pan or a large frying pan and fry the chicken or pork until golden. Remove with a slatted spoon and set aside. Add the onion and red pepper to the pan and fry until soft. Add the stock, garlic, saffron and paprika, return the chicken/pork to the pan, bring to the boil and then turn down the heat. Simmer for 5 minutes, add the rice, tomato and peas and simmer gently for 15 minutes or so, adding more stock if the rice dries out before it is tender, and stirring from time to time. When the rice is nearly tender, add the white fish, prawns, mussels, artichoke hearts and parsley. Season and simmer for 5 minutes and serve.

(**Note:** The rice grains should be tender but not mushy – paella is a little drier than risotto. If using fresh mussels in their shells, discard any that have not opened when ready to serve.)

PASTA AND TUNA BAKE

(Serves 2, ▲▲▲▲▲▲▲▲▲▲▲ per portion)

125 g (4½ oz) [dry weight] pasta shapes (e.g., macaroni)
175 g (6 oz) tuna in brine, drained
1 tbsp chopped parsley
2 black olives, stoned and chopped (optional)
2 tomatoes, skinned, de-seeded and chopped
2 spring onions, finely chopped
1 quantity (2 portions) Cheese Sauce (see recipe on page 89)
25 g (1 oz) brown breadcrumbs
25 g (1 oz) reduced-fat Cheddar cheese, grated
Little salt if necessary

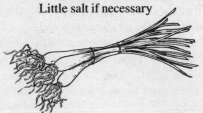

Boil the pasta until just tender (about 10 minutes); drain and keep warm. Arrange the tuna, pasta, parsley, olives, tomato and onion in 2 gratin dishes (or 1 baking dish if preferred) and pour sauce over. Top with the breadcrumbs and cheese and bake at 400°F/200°C/Gas mark 6 for 20 minutes until top is golden.

Variation
● Use 100 g (3½ oz) pasta and 25 g (1 oz) cooked cannellini (white Italian) beans or butter beans

DESSERTS

FRUIT-FILLED FLANS
(Serves 2, ▲▲▲▲ per portion)

2 tsp sunflower oil or use Fry Light spray
2 oblong sheets filo pastry (thawed if frozen)
1 kiwifruit or small peach
1 small banana
50 g (2 oz) grapes or strawberries, halved
1 small orange
Dash of lemon juice
50 ml (2 fl oz) orange juice
1 tsp arrowroot
2 tsp low-sugar apricot jam
4 tsp Greek yogurt

Preheat oven to 400°F/200°C/Gas mark 6. Brush or spray 2 individual flan tins or foil pudding tins with oil very lightly.

Cut the sheets of filo into four each and layer them together, trimming the edges into a rough round. Brush the top layer with oil or spray as before. Line the two containers with the filo layers and press in gently. Bake for a few minutes until golden brown. Remove from oven, leave them to cool, then remove from containers.

Meanwhile prepare the fruit by peeling, deseeding and chopping as necessary into bite-sized pieces. Toss the banana pieces in the lemon juice to prevent them browning. Mix the orange juice, arrowroot and jam together and heat in a small saucepan until the mixture becomes a sauce. Arrange the fruit in the filo cases and pour the sauce over. Top each with the yogurt to serve.

Variation
● Substitute other fruit according to your preference and what is in season

FRUIT PANCAKES WITH CREAMY SAUCE

(Serves 2, ▲▲▲ per portion)

Pancakes (makes 2)
40 g (1½ oz) plain flour
½ size-3 egg, beaten
40 ml (1½ fl oz) skimmed milk mixed with
25 ml (1 fl oz) water
Salt
1 tsp oil *or* Fry Light spray to coat frying pan

Fruit filling
75 g (3 oz) strawberries, sliced, *or* raspberries
50 g (2 oz) peach, sliced, *or* kiwifruit, sliced
1 tsp fructose

Topping
3 tbsp fromage frais
1 tbsp skimmed milk
1 tsp fructose
or
3 tbsp Greek yogurt

Prepare the fruit filling by mixing the fruit with the fructose and leave in fridge until needed. Prepare the topping by mixing together the fromage frais, milk and fructose and leave in fridge until needed.

To make the pancakes, beat together in a small mixing bowl the flour, egg, skimmed milk mixture and salt until smooth. Brush a small non-stick frying pan with the oil, or spray it with Fry Light, and heat the pan until very hot. Add half the pancake mixture, swirling it around to coat evenly. Cook the pancake on high heat until golden on the underside. With a large spatula, turn the pancake over and cook the other side for a few seconds.

Turn out on to a warmed serving plate, fill with the fruit mixture and fold or roll up. Top with the topping or the Greek yogurtand serve.

(**Note:** If you are cooking for two and don't want to waste half an egg, make up double the quantity of pancake mixture and freeze half either as batter or as the made-up pancakes.)

BLACKCURRANT CHEESECAKE
(Serves 8, ▲▲▲ per portion)

40 g (1¹/₂ oz) low-fat spread
8 digestive biscuits, crushed
300 g (11 oz) blackcurrants, topped and tailed
1 rounded tbsp fructose
300 g (11 oz) fromage frais
1 tsp lemon juice
1¹/₂ sachets of gelatine
150 ml (5¹/₂ fl oz) low-fat Bio yogurt

Melt the low-fat spread and mix the crushed biscuits into it in a bowl. Press the biscuit mixture firmly into the base of a 7-inch (18 cm), loose-bottomed cake tin.

Simmer the blackcurrants with a very little water for a few minutes, then stir in the fructose. Whiz the blackcurrants, fromage frais and lemon juice in a blender. Dissolve the gelatine in a little very hot water and stir it and the yogurt very thoroughly into the blackcurrant mixture. Spoon the mixture evenly over the biscuit base. Chill until set.

Variation
● Try using strawberries instead of blackcurrants

THE FREESTYLE PLAN

For long-term slimming, you can use the pyramid below and the appendix at the back of the book to devise meals and recipes of your own.

All you do is make up your day's diet aiming, as near as possible, for these triangles: **9 Starch, 7 Fruit and Vegetable, 5 Protein, 3 Fat,** and **1 Sugar and Alcohol**.

The foods in the appendix are listed together in these groups to make life easier, and you can read Step Six for more information on building a programme from these lists.

I suggest that to start with you draw up some blank triangles like this one below and cross off the triangles in each level as you eat the food they represent. The total number of triangles in this pyramid is 25, giving you a daily total of approximately 1,250 calories. If this amount is too little for you, you can always add extra triangles, but try to keep them in proportion so you retain the pyramid shape to your diet.

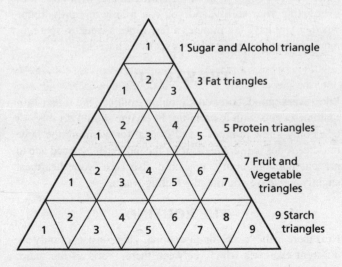

CHAPTER FOUR

Get Moving!

The Slim for Life Flexi-Programme

The strength/tone and stretch Flexi-Programme that follows is the simplest-ever way to get – or maintain – basic body strength, tone and suppleness.

It is totally flexible in terms of fitness ability and available time. You can begin it, however unfit you are, with no fear of over-taxing your ability, and you can follow this programme whether you have ten minutes a few times a week to spare, or much more (up to thirty minutes six times a week).

THE WARM-UP

Like every good body-conditioning routine, the Flexi-Programme begins with a warm-up. Everyone should do this – it takes only a few minutes – and is vital for warming the large muscle groups to prepare them for the movements ahead and to prevent possible injury. It should also raise your heartbeat slightly and leave you literally feeling warm.

THE ROUTINE

Next there is the 'core' toning routine. This consists of only six different exercises which, between them, work all the major muscle groups of your body. You don't *need* to do lots of different exercises for each part of the body, so I've cut this routine right down to the basics to make it easy to follow and simple to do.

Each of the six exercises has three different levels of ability. Level One is the easiest, and everyone should begin on this level. Level Two is a slightly harder version of the basic Level One move and should be attempted when the Level One move becomes easy. Level Three is harder still and should be attempted when you have mastered the Level Two move.

THE COOL-DOWN STRETCHES

The last part of the programme contains a set of gentle stretches, which also act as a cool-down, leaving you feeling refreshed and relaxed. Since your body will be well warmed up after the core exercise routine you will find it easier to stretch it into the movements.

There are nine stretches covering all parts of the body, and doing them for a few minutes at the end of the routine will ensure that you have no aches and pains the next day, as well as increasing your body's flexibility.

HOW MUCH TIME SHOULD YOU SPEND ON THE FLEXI-PROGRAMME?

The complete routine (including warm-up and stretches) should take a minimum of ten minutes. This is based on three minutes each for the warm-up and cool-down stretches, and four minutes to complete *one set* of each of the six core exercises. *One set* means each exercise is repeated *eight times* in a slow and controlled manner.

I suggest that everyone starts with this ten-minute, one-set routine, at least for the first week or two. After that, you can simply stick with ten minutes per session, gradually increasing the difficulty of the programme as you get fitter by moving through Levels Two and Three, and by improving the positions in which you hold the cool-down stretches.

Alternatively, you can increase the number of sets you do of the core exercises. To do this you repeat an exercise eight times for one set, then stop and take a rest for ten to fifteen seconds before doing another set of eight. Doing the whole routine with *two sets* will take you approximately fifteen minutes, with *three* sets, about twenty minutes, and so on. You can do as many sets as you like as long as you build up gradually and don't attempt too much too soon.

Obviously, the more sets you do and the sooner you move through the levels to the harder exercises, the quicker you will build muscle strength and tone.

HOW OFTEN SHOULD YOU DO THE ROUTINE?

The minimum I recommend for acceptable results is three times a week of the basic ten-minute routine. That amounts to just half an hour a week! However, if you choose to do the routine more often than that, again, you will become fitter more quickly. You can do it up to six times a week if you wish, but initially I suggest you start with three times a week of the basic ten-minute routine and see how you go.

Eventually, you can build up to thirty minutes six times a week, if you like, or you can simply do the ten-minute routine three times a week indefinitely for basic strength and tone maintenance. It may be that some weeks you do more, other weeks less. Always remember that a little activity done regularly is much, much better than doing none at all.

To sum up these are the ways you can tailor the Flexi-Programme to suit your needs:

1. There are three levels of ability for each of the six core exercises (Level One, easy; Level Two, harder; Level Three, hardest). You do the one that suits your current fitness level and move to the next one as you improve.

2. You do from one to five sets of each exercise depending on how much time you have. One set is eight repetitions, and the ten-minute routine contains one set of each core exercise. Five sets will increase the total time for the whole routine to thirty minutes.

3. You decide how many times a week you do the routine. A ten-minute routine three times a week performed regularly will achieve results.

TIPS TO HELP YOU

- Exercise in a warm room and wear comfortable, non-restrictive clothing.
- Make sure the floor is not too hard and, if it is not carpeted, use a good, thick, non-slip mat to exercise on.
- Don't exercise if you are ill.
- Breathe comfortably throughout.
- Concentrate as you do the movements; do them in a slow and controlled way.
- Move into a stretch and hold the position, rather than doing repeated bounces.
- If you are doing the programme properly – and moving up through the levels when you are ready – the routine should make you feel that your body is working, but there should be no pain. If you reach a stage during the core routine when the muscle you are exercising begins to shake, then stop – you have done enough.
- When doing the stretches, you should feel a pleasant, warm sensation in the muscle(s) being stretched, but not a nasty burning. It is important to try to breathe deeply and relax into the stretch. You may then be able to achieve a bigger stretch without strain. Stop if any muscle hurts.

> *Do not begin this programme until you have read the preceding pages and understand what you should be doing.*

The Flexi warm-up

Starting Position

- Stand with your feet slightly apart, knees relaxed and pointing in the same direction as your toes. Keep your back straight, stomach pulled in and shoulders back and down.

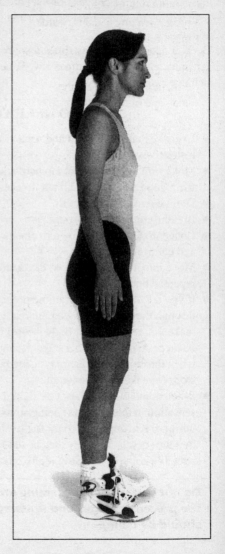

1. Shoulder rolls

- Lift the shoulders up and back, then down and forwards in a circular motion.
- Repeat 8 times, then reverse the action in a forwards direction 8 times. Feel the neck and upper back loosen up.

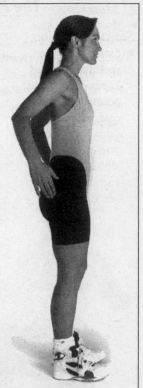

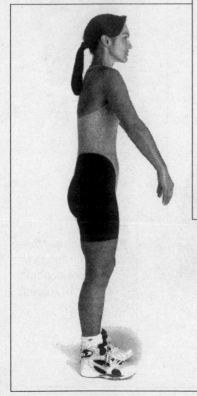

2. Marching

- March on the spot, pumping your arms backwards and forwards for 1 minute. Start with low marches and gradually raise knees higher and higher until you are breathing deeply.

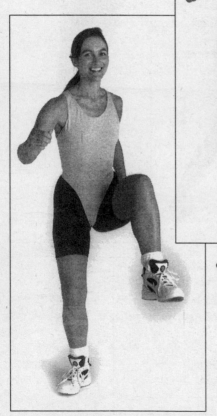

- Continue marching but with legs in a wide position for a further 10 seconds.

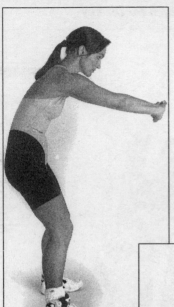

3. *Low-back release*
- Keep the feet in the wide position, extend your arms forwards at shoulder level and link hands loosely. Everything else is in the starting position.
- Let the knees bend a little further as you curl the back into a letter C-shape and pull the stomach in. Hold for 10 seconds. Release and repeat.

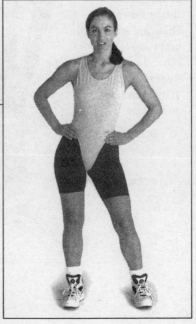

4. *Hip circles*
- In the starting position, but with feet wide, imagine you have a hula hoop and circle your hips very slowly a few times, first in a clockwise direction and then in an anti-clockwise direction.

5. *Side to side sway and reach for the sky*

- With the feet still in the wide position shift your weight from side to side, bending the knee of the leg you are moving as you come up on the toes of the opposite foot. As you move to the right, lift your left arm up and across, palm facing forwards, changing arms as you sway to the other side.
- Repeat 20 times, 10 to each side alternately.

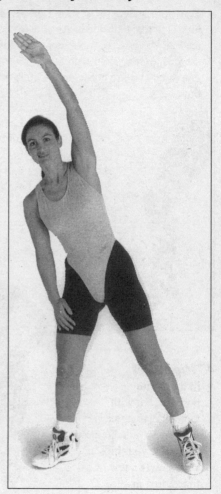

6. Step touch with arm swings

- Take your weight on to your left foot and bring your right foot in to touch beside it. As you do so, swing your arms to the left. Reverse the movement by taking your right foot to the side, putting your weight on it and bringing the left foot in to touch beside it. Swing the arms across at the same time.

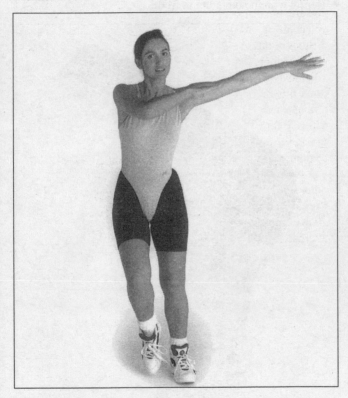

- Repeat 20 times in all, 10 to each side with the arms flowing from side to side. You can clap if you like as the arms swing to the side.

7. *Hamstring and calf stretch*

- Bend your left knee and take your right leg out in front of
  you. Keeping your right leg straight, lean over it, bending
  from the hips and supporting your body with your hands on
  your left thigh. Feel the stretch in the back of the right thigh.
  Lift your right toes to add a mid-calf stretch. Hold for 10
  seconds.
- Repeat with the other leg in front.

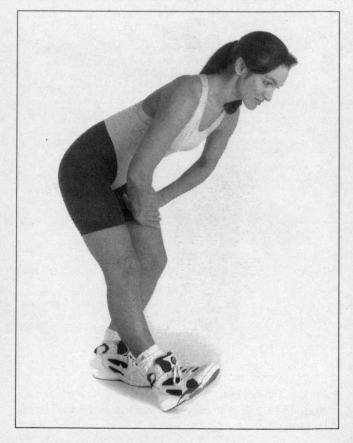

8. *Quadricep stretch*

- Stand in the starting position and hold on to a chair or stool with your left hand (or place your left hand against a wall to support yourself). Grasp the middle part of your right foot (or your right heel) with your right hand and bring it towards your bottom. Feel the front of your thigh stretch out. Hold for 8 seconds.
- Repeat with the other leg.

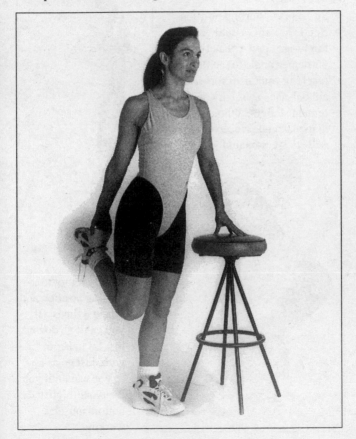

Strength and Tone

Now you are warmed up you can begin the strength and tone exercises. Remember, if you are new to this routine, start on Level One for each of the six exercises.

1. SQUATS: FOR THIGHS AND BOTTOM

Level One
- Stand in the starting position.
- Bend your knees until your thighs are approximately at a 45-degree angle to the floor, reaching your arms forwards to aid balance. Your back should remain straight, although at a diagonal angle since your hips will stick out behind you.

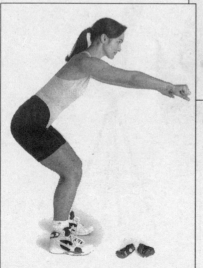

- Slowly return to the starting position and repeat 8 times. (If you can't go down that far to begin with, just go as far as you can until you feel your thigh and bottom muscles working.)

Level Two

- As Level One but this time squatting down further until your thighs are almost parallel to the floor, if possible. Do not go any lower than this point.
- Repeat 8 times slowly for one set.

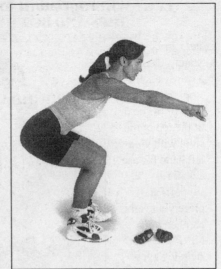

Level Three

- As Level Two but adding some arm strengthening work. Pick up your handweights (or cans of beans). Keep your elbows by your sides and bring your hands towards your shoulders as you squat down. Return hands to your sides as you raise up.
- Repeat 8 times slowly for one set.

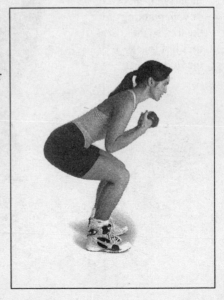

2. LEG SWEEPS: FOR OUTER THIGHS, HIPS AND BOTTOM

Level One

- Stand side on to a sturdy chair or stool. Hold the back of the chair or the top of the stool with your left hand (or use a wall for support) and place your right hand on your hip. Place your right leg a few inches in front of you, pointing the toes so the toes just touch the floor.

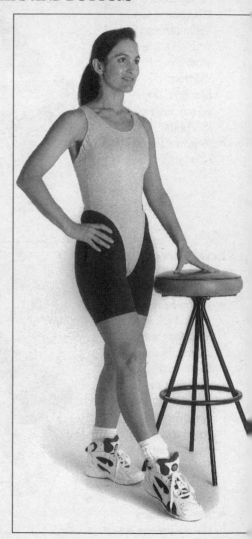

- In a sweeping motion, bring your right leg around to the right and then to the back of you, all the time keeping the toes in contact with the floor to aid balance. Reverse the movement to sweep the leg around to the front again, and repeat 8 times.

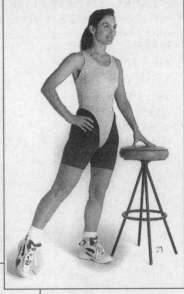

- Turn around and repeat 8 times with your left leg for a complete set.

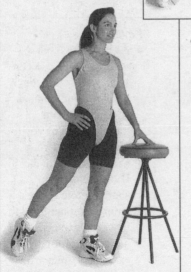

Level Two

- Use an exercise
rubber band or a
tied Dyna-Band.
Place the band
around your
ankles. Perform the
exercise 8 times
with each leg,
sweeping the leg
around as before.

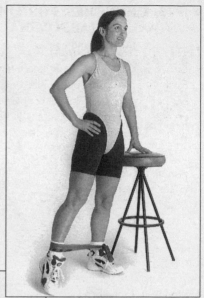

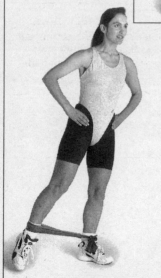

Level Three

- As Level Two but
without support. Keep
your body stabilized by
holding your stomach
back and bottom
muscles tight as you
perform the exercise.
(You can also tie the
Dyna-Band into a
shorter circle or use a
stronger rubber band to
make the exercise
harder.) Perform the
exercise 8 times with
each leg.

3. CRUNCHES: FOR THE STOMACH (ABDOMINALS)

Level One (Basic crunch)

- Lie on your back with your knees bent, feet flat on the floor. Rest your hands on your thighs, or have them behind the base of your head. (This latter arm position makes the crunch a little more difficult but helps support the weight of the head and may prevent neck ache.)

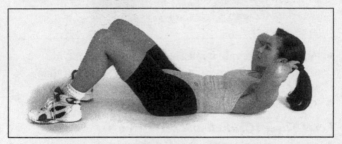

- Slowly raise the head and shoulder blades off the floor, using the abdominal muscles to make a curling action and bringing the rib cage towards the thighs.
- Lower, and repeat 8 times for one set.

Level Two (Reverse curl)

- Lie flat, bring your knees into the chest with ankles crossed and feet relaxed down towards the thighs. Have your hands behind your head.

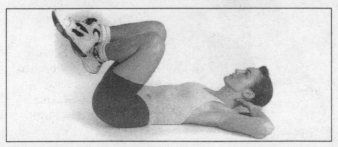

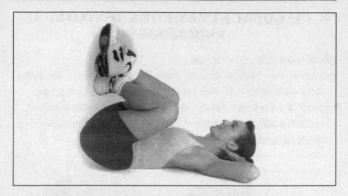

- Pull in the abdominal muscles so that the hips move towards your rib cage – it is a rolling action rather than a pushing-up action. Be careful not to swing the legs.
- Repeat 8 times for one set.

Level Three (Crunch and reverse curl)
- Start in the same position as Level Two.
- Combine the movements of Levels One and Two by lifting your head and shoulders off the floor, bringing your rib cage towards your knees as you also use the abdominal muscles to roll the hips in.

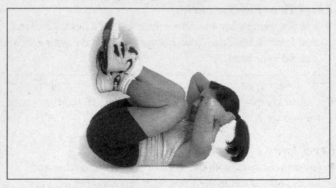

- Repeat 8 times for one set.

4. DIAGONAL CURLS: FOR THE STOMACH (ABDOMINALS)

Level One

- Lie on your back with your knees bent, feet flat on the floor and hands behind your head.
- Keeping your hips flat on the floor, take the right shoulder over towards the left knee – you can lead with the right elbow. The other elbow should be on the floor to give you support as you lift. Lower, and reverse sides.

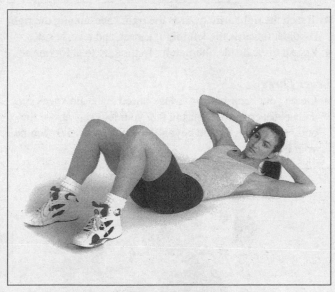

- Continue repeating to each side alternately, 16 times in total for one set.

Level Two

- Lie on your back with the soles of your feet together and knees relaxed out to the sides, your left hand behind your head.

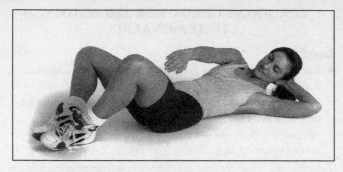

- Reach the right arm towards the right knee, aiming the right shoulder towards the left thigh. Lower, and reverse sides.
- Repeat to each side alternately, 16 times in total for one set.

Level Three

- Lie on your back with your legs raised in the air, knees bent and ankles crossed, ensuring that your legs stay above the body and do not extend beyond it. Place your hands behind your head.

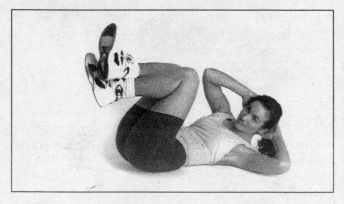

- Take the right shoulder across towards the outside of the left thigh, leading with both elbows. Lower, and reverse sides.
- Repeat to each side alternately, 16 times in total for one set.

5. PRESS-UPS: FOR UPPER BODY, CHEST AND ARMS

Level One

- Start by kneeling on all fours with thighs at right angles to the floor. Your back is straight and your stomach pulled in. Ensure that your wrists are in line with your shoulders and that your fingers are pointing forwards.

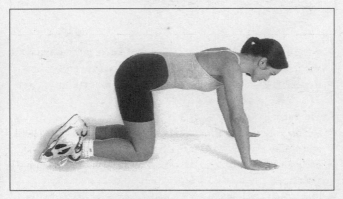

- Lower the chest towards the floor. Go as far as you can, then slowly return to the starting position.

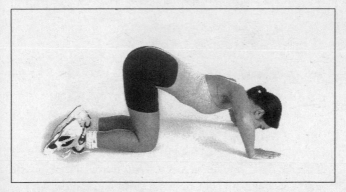

- Repeat 8 times for one set.

Level Two

● Kneel as before but with your hands and shoulders further forwards and your ankles lifted so that your bottom is halfway to the floor.

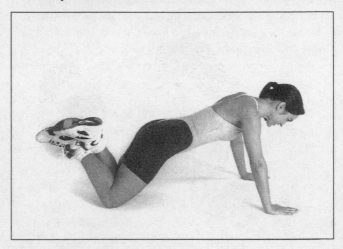

● Lower and raise the chest 8 times as before.

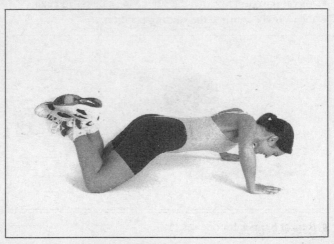

Level Three

- Start with your legs straight, hips slightly lifted and wrists in line with your shoulders.

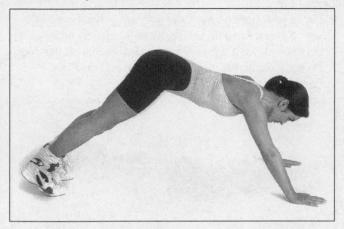

- Slowly lower your chest to the floor, then raise up. Keep your back straight, hips slightly lifted and stomach in. This is a full press-up.

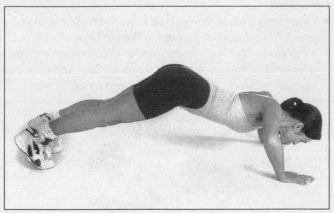

- Repeat 8 times.

6. BACK EXTENSIONS: FOR THE LOWER BACK

Level One
- Lie on your front with arms by your sides, hands resting on your bottom. Keeping your hips and legs firmly anchored to the floor, slowly raise your head and shoulders off the floor. Do not look up, but keep your face towards the floor. Lower, and repeat.

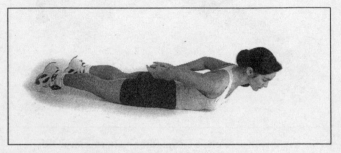

- Repeat 8 times for one set.

Level Two
- Lie on your front with your right hand under your head and your left hand extended along the floor in front of you.
- Keep your lower body on the floor and lift your left arm and your head, keeping your face towards the floor and your neck long. Slowly return to the floor, and repeat 8 times.

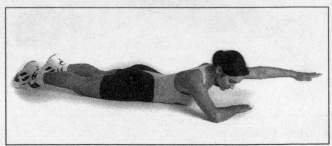

- Change sides and perform the exercise 8 times, lifting the right arm.

Level Three

- As Level Two, but as the left arm lifts, raise the right leg, still ensuring the hips stay in contact with the floor. Slowly return to the floor, and repeat 8 times.

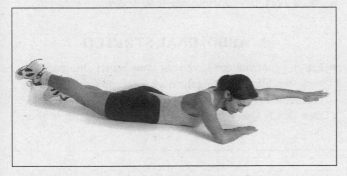

- Change sides, and repeat 8 times. (This exercise also strengthens the muscles of the bottom.)

Stretch and Cool-Down

Hold each of the following stretches for a minimum of 10 seconds. As you get used to the stretches you can stay in them for 30 seconds each. As you become more supple you will be able to develop a better stretch. The photos are only a guide, so don't worry if you cannot reach as far to start with – muscles that have not been worked for a while take time to develop flexibility.

1. ABDOMINAL STRETCH

- Lie on your front and have your arms bent, palms beside your shoulders. Keeping the neck long and forearms in contact with the floor, raise the chest and shoulders. Hold, then slowly lower. Feel this stretch along the front of your body.

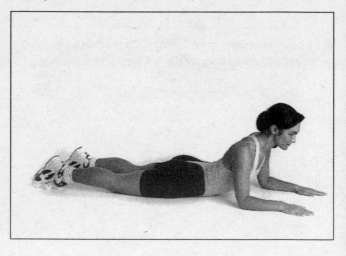

2. FRONT THIGH (QUADRICEP) STRETCH

● Lying on your front, hold the middle of your right foot or its
  heel with your right hand and bring it in towards your hips.
  Make sure you keep the knees together and your hips in
  contact with the floor. (If, initially, you are not able to reach
  your foot, wrap a towel around the foot and hold both ends
  to bring the foot in towards the body.) Hold, then release.

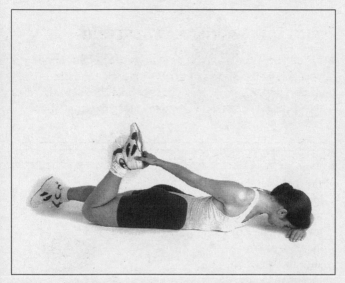

● Repeat with the other foot. You will feel this stretch along
  the front of your thigh.

3. BACK STRETCH SEQUENCE

This sequence will give you a pleasant stretch all along the back.

- Start on all fours with hands under your shoulders, and arch your back like a cat. Hold, then slowly return to a flat back.

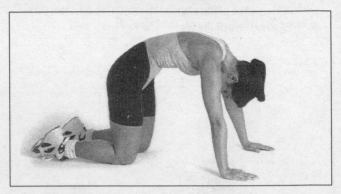

- From all fours, slowly lower the hips down on to the calves, then lower the chest to the floor as you slide the hands forwards. Hold.

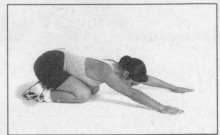

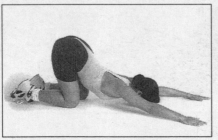

- To increase this stretch, raise the hips off the calves. You may also be able to slide the fingers further forwards.

4. BACK OF THIGH (HAMSTRING) STRETCH

- Lie on your back with both knees bent and feet flat on the floor.
- With one hand on your left calf, bring the left knee in towards your chest, then slowly straighten the left leg until you feel a stretch at the back of the thigh. Hold, then bring the leg in and return the foot to the floor.

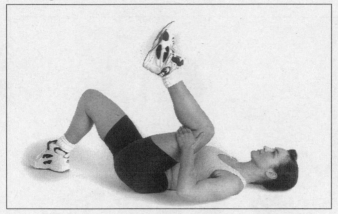

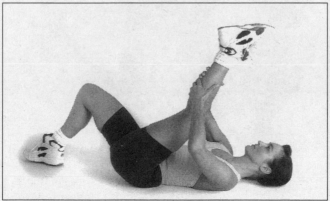

- Repeat with the other leg.

5. INNER THIGH STRETCH

● Sitting up (on a mat or a towel if this is more comfortable),
place the soles of the feet together and let the knees fall to
the sides. Hold loosely on to the calves or feet and let your
elbows press gently on to your knees, easing them towards
the floor. You will feel the stretch along the inner thighs. As
you progress, your knees will come nearer to the floor.

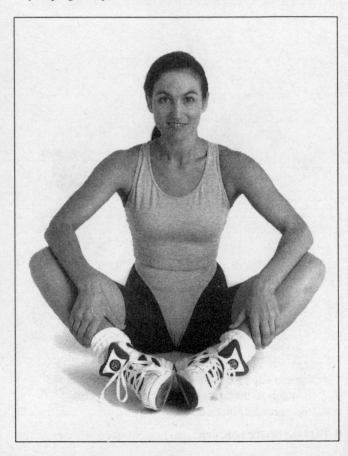

6. OUTER THIGH AND HIP STRETCH

- Sit with your left leg extended in front of you, bend the right leg and cross it over the left. Hold your right leg with your left arm and gently ease the knee into your body. You will feel a stretch along the right hip and outer thigh.

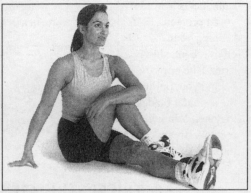

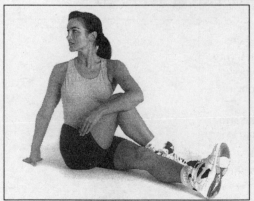

- You can add a torso stretch by turning your head and shoulders to the right. Hold, then slowly uncurl.
- Repeat on the other side.

The next two stretches can also be performed standing.

7. CHEST STRETCH

- Sit with your legs in a comfortable position for you and your back straight. Link hands behind your back and, keeping your elbows bent, slowly extend the arms behind you, pulling the shoulder blades together. You will feel this stretch through your chest.

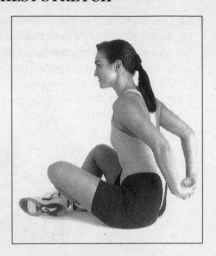

8. TRICEP STRETCH

- Still sitting comfortably, bend your left arm, trying to keep the elbow close to your head. Apply gentle pressure to the arm to increase the stretch. Hold.
- Repeat on the other side.

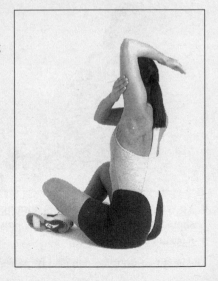

9. LONG BODY STRETCH

● Lie on your back with your knees bent and your arms
   outstretched on the floor above your head. If you have a
   tight chest or tight shoulders you will find it impossible to
   get your arms and your back on the floor. If that is the case,
   carefully raise your back off the floor so that you can get
   your arms on the floor, then slowly press your back into the
   floor again, concentrating on keeping your arms flat for as
   long as possible. Over the weeks you will gradually be able
   to stretch out flat from your bottom up to your fingertips.
   As you stretch, you will feel your stomach really flattening
   towards your spine and your chest expanding.

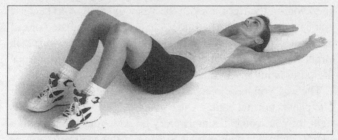

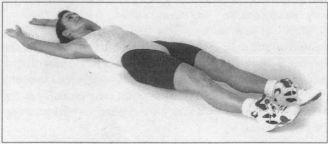

● After holding this position for a minimum of 10 seconds,
   stretch out both legs, one at a time, until your whole body is
   flat on the floor. Hold this long body stretch for a further 10
   seconds. Sometimes I hold it for up to 3 minutes!

CHAPTER FIVE

Consolidate

From the moment you first picked up this book, you have been learning not just how to get slim, but how to *stay* slim for the rest of your life.

The ideas, thoughts, motivations and the insights and knowledge that this book has helped you to gain are those that will keep you on the right track in the years to come. And because you haven't been 'on a diet' as such, we have eliminated one of the greatest problems that most people meet when they do reach target weight at the end of a diet – how to get back to 'normal life' after being in 'dieting life'.

The way you have been eating to lose weight on the *Slim for Life* plan *is* normal eating. Once you are at the weight that feels right for you, you can simply carry on with your life, and your swops, and your new way of looking at things. There will be only one real change – *you can eat more*.

When you were losing weight, however slowly, you had to create a calorie deficit so that your body used its own fat stores for energy. Now that you no longer need a deficit, you will need enough food to maintain your new body weight, and this will inevitably mean eating more. So you just carry on eating in the pyramid fashion – or as near as you can get to it – but increasing the portion sizes.

Easy ways to weight maintenance

To give you an example of how simple the change is, many of you will have been eating, at least some of the time, around

25 triangles a day during your slimming campaign, using a pyramid-style diet like this:

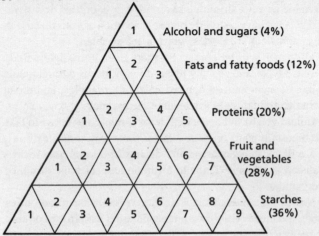

On your maintenance programme, you should be able to increase that to *at least* 36 triangles a day (remember, each triangle is worth 50 calories), which would look like this:

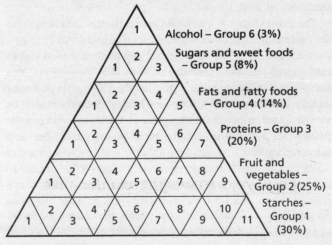

You can have 11 starch triangles a day; 9 fruit and vegetable; 7 protein; 5 fats; 3 sugars, and 1 alcohol. This balance is almost the same as your slimming pyramid, except on this new pyramid you can have a slightly higher proportion of your diet as fat, sugar and alcohol calories, which is reasonable.

Most men will be able to eat more than 36 triangles. Body weights, types and activity levels do vary, but as a rough guide I suggest men start on approximately 48 triangles, adding an extra two triangles to each level of the pyramid.

Unless you have been a long-term slimmer and chose to take the 'freestyle plan' on page 105 for more long-term flexibility, you will have been using the meal suggestions and recipes included in Chapter Three to form the basis of your slimming programme.

Now, to maintain your weight, you will want to add other foods and create your own menus. In order to help you do this, I have listed all the most popular food items with their triangle rating in the Food Charts starting on page 148. By using this list, you will find it easy to build your own pyramid-style diet, adding extra foods, creating your own recipes and using new foods as you wish.

The Food Charts group foods in exactly the same way as in the 36-triangle pyramid on the facing page so that you can easily see which 'tier' of the pyramid any particular food comes into and so tell how your day's pyramid is shaping up. You don't need to be precise – for instance, by always eating exactly 11 triangles of starchy foods a day. In fact, it would be very difficult to be absolutely precise. I'd like you to use the 36-triangle pyramid as nothing more than a guide. But as a matter of interest, it would be good now and then to have a day when you do check out more precisely what you're eating. To do this, draw up a blank 36-triangle pyramid and cross off each triangle when you have eaten food to that triangle value on each level.

TIPS TO KEEP YOU SLIM FOR LIFE

- Remember, you are in control of what you put into your mouth – no-one else. It's your choice, but don't be obsessive or rigid in your control. Enjoy your food and feel relaxed about food. But never be afraid to say 'no' to the things you don't want.
- Don't feel guilty about enjoying hearty, tasty meals and don't feel guilty if occasionally you eat something that afterwards you wish you hadn't. Slim people eat all kinds of high- and low-calorie foods and stay slim because they take a 'swings and roundabouts' approach. You can do that too because you *are* a slim person.
- If you find difficulty in coping with certain areas of your eating habits, go back to Chapter Two and work through this or these areas again. There is no time limit on learning new ways to deal with your food intake.
- Remember, that you aren't perfect – no-one is.
- Be happy with sustainable goals. Don't try for too low a maintenance weight. Don't expect to look perfect – no-one does.
- Stay motivated and keep active.
- Listen to your body. It will let you know when you really are hungry.
- Eat slowly and enjoy your food.
- Remember, food isn't the most important thing in your life, even if it once was. Food is fuel to help you to a healthy body. You don't live to eat; you eat to live.

Write a list here of all the things that are important to you now:

....

....

....

....

STAY MOTIVATED

It is important to remind yourself now and then of all the ways your body, your mind and your life have improved since you began to lose weight. Do you feel many of these benefits now? Which things can you work on to consolidate your success? What did you hope to achieve once you were slim? Isn't it time to start work on those ambitions now?

If everything is going on much as before, except that you feel slimmer and fitter and you like your body better – well, that's terrific too.

But in that case, can I offer you a motivator that will help everyone achieve long-term slimness. I would like you to get involved in a new campaign of mine – one that would ultimately result in me being rendered out of a job. I hope that, with your help, obesity in this country will eventually be wiped out, and that ill health through overweight and poor diet will be a thing of the past.

Sounds amazing? Well, maybe, but with your help, it could work. Turn to page 147 to see what you can do.

KEEP ACTIVE

People who keep themselves physically active find that they can eat plenty without putting on weight. If you combine a sensible pyramid-style of eating with a reasonable amount of activity, then you have the perfect way to control your weight for the rest of your life.

You can continue with the activity programme in Chapter Four, varying the amount you do from week to week according to what suits you.

To maintain fitness (as opposed to improving) most experts agree that two to three aerobic sessions and two strength/tone/flexibility sessions a week are all that's needed to keep you in shape.

But perhaps the single most important thing you can do to help maintain your new weight is to burn up extra calories each day by keeping as active as you can *outside* the confines of a formal exercise session. Your body needs to be used. Sitting around for most of the day and moving occasionally from bed to chair to car to desk to sofa to bed is not enough.

Give your body the attention it deserves throughout the day. All you need to do is to be aware of your body and to return a little to how your life might have been before TV, cars and labour-saving devices. Remember, every time you say 'yes' to a modern convenience that saves your body from moving or working, you're doing it a disfavour. Here are some ideas on getting more activity and movement into your everyday life:

- Think 'outdoors' as often as possible. Cycle or walk when you can (often it will be just as quick as waiting for a bus that never comes, or finding somewhere to park the car). Make the most of local facilities such as parks and nature trails.
- If you have a garden, spend more time in it. Gardening can be an absorbing and not too expensive hobby that anyone can enjoy.
- To give walking more of a purpose if you need one, consider walking a neighbour's dog or even a neighbour's baby.
- Don't just send your own children out to play – go with them and organise some active games like catch or rounders. Alternatively, take them swimming or roller-skating.
- Find out what clubs there are in your area that you could join. Your local council or library will have details.
- Try to increase the pace at which you do things, e.g., going up stairs, doing housework, carrying shopping, pushing a trolley, walking to work. Doing things faster means speeding up your metabolic rate and burning up more calories.

- Check your posture throughout the day. Whether you are standing or sitting, is your tummy pulled in, your bottom tucked in? Are your shoulders down and relaxed, rather than hunched?

- If you suffer from mid-afternoon sluggishness, don't fall asleep or eat a chocolate bar. If you feel drowsy or lack concentration during the day, a high-sugar, quickly absorbed snack will only end up making you feel worse. Instead, take a five-minute activity break: running up stairs or walking round the room or garden will put your body and brain back in good working order.

- Don't stay in bed longer than necessary to give you a refreshing sleep. Too much sleep can lower metabolism.

- Don't forget to breathe, preferably, good, fresh air. Like a fire, our bodies need oxygen to burn fuel (i.e. to convert food into energy and burn off calories). Whenever you get the chance, stand at an open window and breathe in deeply (not too deeply if you are unused to this as it will make you dizzy, but you'll soon improve). Always breathe calmly but deeply whatever you are doing.

- If you have long periods of standing or sitting, do some movements to get your circulation going again.

While sitting at desk or table: circle ankles; lift lower legs up and down and straighten legs out; flex heels to stretch calves; tighten and release thigh muscles; tighten and release buttock muscles; circle shoulders and gently turn head from left to right; gently pull head down to chest to release neck.

While standing in kitchen waiting for the kettle to boil: support yourself with one hand on work surface and do some leg sweeps (see page 120); stand with feet apart and knees bent and gently swing upper body down until fingers touch floor to release a tight back; clench buttock muscles; put one leg in front of the other and lift front heel off floor several times to exercise calf muscles.

By giving your body a series of mini workouts during the day you are doing a great deal to help keep it toned and supple, as well as burning off calories and preventing a build up of muscle tension.

Well, those are my ideas. I'm sure you can think of more. Write down here ten things you can do to build more activity into your life. Pick the ones that appeal to you from my list or choose your own.

Remember, if you want your body to be slim and to give you long-lasting, non-stop, uncomplaining service, treat it well, use it. You can't replace it!

Now see what you can change!

Over the last twenty years I have helped hundreds of thousands of people to lose weight through my books, magazine and newspaper columns. I hope that you are now one of them. But wouldn't it have been better if you hadn't had to slim because you hadn't put on the excess weight in the first place?

As we discussed earlier, there are many reasons why people put on too much weight. Most of those reasons can be summed up as 'outside influences' that made you eat too much of the wrong things and take too little exercise.

In order for you to lose weight I had to show you how to take control of your own body and cope with – or ignore – outside influences. Now that you are slim, you can go one better. Isn't it time to see what influence *you* can have on *others*? Not only on the people you know, but on the people and organisations who make the decisions that help keep us, as a nation, fat?

If we all campaigned determinedly enough, within a few generations we could have overweight, obesity, and the misery and ill health that they cause, licked for good.

THE FOOD CHARTS

The charts will help you to follow a pyramid-style way of eating to maintain your new weight. The foods are grouped in the same way as in the 36-triangle pyramid that forms the 'blueprint' for your maintenance diet (see page 141).

They are:

Group 1:   Starches group, including breads, crispbreads and bakery items; breakfast cereals; rice, grains and pasta; potatoes.
Aim for: approximately 11 triangles a day from this group.

Group 2:   Fruit and vegetables group, including all fresh fruit; all fresh and frozen vegetables; fruit and vegetable juices; dried fruits and pulses.
Aim for: approximately 9 triangles a day from this group.

Group 3:   Protein group, including low- to medium-fat cheeses; eggs; fish and seafood; low- to medium-fat meats; poultry; low- to medium-fat milk, yogurt and fromage frais products; vegetable proteins.
Aim for: approximately 7 triangles a day from this group.

Group 4:   Fats group, including all fats and oils; oily dressings, nuts and snacks; all savoury high-fat and fried foods.
Aim for: 5 triangles a day from this group.

Group 5:   Sugars and sweet items, including sweets and chocolate; cakes; biscuits and desserts.
Aim for: 3 triangles a day from this group.

Group 6:   Alcohol.
Aim for: 1 triangle a day from this group, or amalgamate with the sugars Group 5, and aim for a total of 4 triangles a day for Groups 5 and 6.

Note: · All triangle values are approximate, not exact – many values have been rounded up or down.

Group 1: Starches

BREADS, CRISPBREADS AND BAKERY ITEMS

All per 25 g (1 oz) unless otherwise stated.

No. of triangles

Bread

Brown, wheatgerm, white or wholemeal, per 40 g (1½ oz) slice from a large loaf, medium cut	2
French bread, brown or white	2
Petit pain, one whole	2
Pitta bread, white, one large	4
Pitta bread, wholemeal, one large	3
Pitta bread, one mini	2
Roll, one average	2½
Bap, one average	3

Crispbreads

Average rye crispbread, one	½
Crisproll, one	½

Bakery items

Crumpet, one	1½
Currant bun, one	3
English muffin, one	3
Malt loaf, 25 g (1 oz) slice	1½
Pancake, one average	2
Scone, one average	3
Teacake, one	3

BREAKFAST CEREALS

All per 25 g (1 oz) unless otherwise stated

All Bran	1½
Bran flakes or corn flakes	2
Fruit 'n' Fibre or muesli	2
Porridge oats, raw weight	2

No. of triangles

Porridge, made up with water, per 200 ml (7 fl oz) bowlful	2
Shredded Wheat, one	2
Weetabix, one	1½

RICE, GRAINS AND PASTA

Bulgar wheat or couscous, dry weight, per 25 g (1 oz)	2
Flour, white, wholemeal, soya or buckwheat, per 25 g (1 oz)	2
Pasta, all types, uncooked weight, per 25 g (1 oz)	2
Pasta, all types, boiled weight, per 100 g (3½ oz)	2
Pearl barley, dry weight, per 25 g (1 oz)	2
Rice, all types, dry weight, per 25 g (1 oz)	2
Rice, all types, boiled weight, per 100 g (3½ oz)	2
Semolina or polenta, dry weight, per 25 g (1 oz)	2

POTATOES

Baked, one average (225 g, 8 oz)	5
Boiled, per 100 g (4 oz)	1½
Mashed with 7 g (¼ oz) low-fat spread, per 100 g (3½ oz)	2½
Instant mashed, per 100 g (3½ oz)	2
Roast, 1 chunk (50 g, 2 oz)	2½
Sweet potato, baked or boiled, per 100 g (4 oz)	2

(for chips and crisps see Group 4)

Group 2: Fruit and vegetables

DRIED FRUITS

All per 25 g (1 oz) unless otherwise stated

Apples, apricots, currants, figs, peaches, stoned prunes, raisins or sultanas	1
Stoned dates	1½

FRESH FRUIT

No. of triangles

All per item unless otherwise stated

Apple, dessert	1
Apple, cooking	1
Apricot, fresh, two	1
Banana, one small	1
Banana, one large	2
Blackberries, per 100 g (3½ oz)	1
Blackcurrants, per 100 g (3½ oz)	1
Cherries, per 100 g (3½ oz)	1
Damsons, per 100 g (3½ oz)	1
Dates, fresh, three	1
Fig, fresh	1
Gooseberries, dessert, per 100 g (3½ oz)	1
Gooseberries, cooking, per 100 g (3½ oz)	½
Grapefruit, one whole	1
Grapes, per 100 g (3½ oz)	1
Kiwifruit	1
Lemon, one whole	½
Lime, one whole	½
Mango	2
Melon, 200 g (7 oz) slice	1
Nectarine	1
Orange	1
Peach	1
Pear, one average	1
Pear, one large	1½
Pineapple, two slices	1
Plum, two dessert	1
Raspberries, per 100 g (3½ oz)	½
Rhubarb, per 100 g (3½ oz) [4 sticks]	½
Satsuma or tangerine	½
Strawberries, per 100 g (3½ oz)	½

FRUIT AND VEGETABLE JUICES

No. of triangles

All per 125 ml (4½ fl oz), average glass

Apple, grape, grapefruit, citrus,
  orange, pineapple or mixed   1
Mixed vegetable or tomato   ½

NUTS

Chestnuts, shelled, per 25 g (1 oz)   1
(for all other nuts see Group 4)

PULSES

Baked beans in tomato sauce,
  canned, per 100 g (3½ oz)   1½
Butter beans, dry weight, per 25 g (1 oz)   1½
Butter beans, boiled or canned, per 100 g (3½ oz)   2
Chick peas, dry weight, per 25 g (1 oz)   2
Chick peas, boiled or canned, per 100 g (3½ oz)   3
Haricot beans, dry weight, per 25 g (1 oz)   1½
Kidney beans, dry weight, per 25 g (1 oz)   1½
Kidney beans, boiled or canned, per 100 g (3½ oz)   2
Lentils, brown or green, dry weight, per 25 g (1 oz) 1½
Lentils, brown or green, boiled, per 100 g (3½ oz)   2
Lentils, red, dry weight, per 25 g (1 oz)   2
Lentils, red, boiled, per 100 g (3 ½ oz)   2
Lentil soup, per 100 ml (3½ fl oz)   2
Split peas, dry weight, per 25 g (1 oz)   1½
Split peas, boiled, per 100 g (3½ oz)   2½

VEGETABLES

All per 100 g (3½ oz), raw or cooked without fat, unless otherwise stated

Artichoke, globe, one whole   1
Artichoke, Jerusalem   ½

	No. of triangles
Asparagus, five spears	1/2
Aubergine	1/2
Avocado, half a medium	4
Beans, broad	1
Beans, French	1
Beans, runner	1/2
Beansprouts	1/2
Beetroot	1
Broccoli	1/2
Brussels sprouts	1/2
Cabbage, all types	1/2
Carrots	1/2
Cauliflower	1/2
Celeriac	1/2
Celery	1/2
Chicory	1/2
Chinese leaves and Pak Choi	1/2
Corn on the cob, one medium	2
Courgettes	1/2
Cucumber	1/2
Leeks	1/2
Lettuce, all types	1/2
Marrow	1/2
Mushrooms	1/2
Mustard and cress	1/2
Onion, one large	1
Onion, one small	1/2
Onion, spring, one bunch	1/2
Parsnip	1
Peas	1
Pepper, green	1/2
Pepper, red or yellow	1
Radish	1/2
Spinach	1/2

	No. of triangles
Swede	1/2
Sweetcorn kernels	2
Tomato, one large	1/2
Turnip	1/2
Watercress	1/2

Group 3: Proteins

CHEESES

Brie, per 25 g (1 oz)	1 1/2
Camembert, per 25 g (1 oz)	1 1/2
Cheddar-style, half-fat, per 25 g (1 oz)	1 1/2
Cottage, per 100 g (3 1/2 oz)	2
Cottage, diet, per 100 g (3 1/2 oz)	1 1/2
Edam, half-fat type, per 25 g (1 oz)	1 1/2
Low-fat soft cheese, e.g., Shape, per 40 g (1 1/2 oz)	1
Mozzarella, per 25 g (1 oz)	1 1/2
Quark low-fat, per 100 g (3 1/2 oz)	2 1/2
Reduced-fat cheese spread, per 25 g (1 oz)	1

EGGS

Size 1 or 2, each	2
Size 3 or 4, each	1 1/2
Size 3 egg, one, dry-fried	2
Size 3 egg, two, scrambled with 7 g (1/4 oz) low-fat spread and dash skimmed milk	4

FISH AND SEAFOOD

Fish

Cod or coley or haddock fillet, per 100 g (3 1/2 oz)	1 1/2
Halibut steak or plaice fillet, per 100 g (3 1/2 oz)	2

	No. of triangles
Haddock, smoked fillet, per 100 g (3½ oz)	2
Herring, grilled, per 100 g (3½ oz)	4
Kipper, grilled, per 100 g (3½ oz)	4
Monkfish, per 100 g (3½ oz)	1½
Pilchards in tomato sauce, per 100 g (3½ oz)	3
Salmon, fresh fillet, per 100 g (3½ oz)	4
Salmon, canned, drained, per 100 g (3½ oz)	3
Salmon, smoked, per 50 g (2 oz)	1½
Trout, rainbow fillet, per 100 g (3½ oz)	3
Tuna steak, fresh, per 100 g (3½ oz)	3
Tuna canned in brine, drained, per 100 g (3½ oz)	2
Tuna canned in oil, drained, per 100 g (3½ oz)	2½
Fishcake, one, grilled	2
Fish fingers, one, grilled	1
Fish, frozen crumbed portion, baked or grilled, one	4

Seafood

All per 100 g (3½ oz), shelled or dressed weight

Crab	2½
Prawns	2
Mussels	2
Scallops	2
Squid	1½

MEAT AND POULTRY

All per 100 g (3½ oz) unless otherwise stated

Meat

Beef, extra-lean, minced	4
Beef, steak, no visible fat	4
Beef, topside, roast	3
Beef, roast rib, including fat	5
Beef, roast rib, fat removed	4
Beefburger, lean, grilled, 1 × 50 g (2 oz)	2

	No. of triangles
Corned beef	4
Ham, extra-lean	2$\frac{1}{2}$
Kidneys, lamb's, each	1
Lamb, leg, roast, lean only	4
Lamb chop, extra-lean, trimmed, grilled, one	3
Liver, grilled	3$\frac{1}{2}$
Pork, roast, lean only	3$\frac{1}{2}$
Pork fillet, raw	3$\frac{1}{2}$
Rabbit, flesh only	3
Sausages, low-fat, grilled, per chipolata	1
Veal	2

Poultry and game

Chicken, meat only (no skin)	3
Chicken, roast, meat and skin	4
Duck, roast, lean only	4
Turkey, roast or fillet	2
Venison	4

MILK, YOGURT AND FROMAGE FRAIS

Milk, semi-skimmed, per 100 ml (3$\frac{1}{2}$ fl oz)	1
Milk, skimmed, per 150 ml (5$\frac{1}{2}$ fl oz)	1
Milk, soya, per 150 ml (5$\frac{1}{2}$ fl oz)	1
Yogurt, diet fruit, per tub	1
Yogurt, fruit, low-fat, per 100 ml (3$\frac{1}{2}$ fl oz)	2
Yogurt, Greek cow's, strained, per 100 ml (3$\frac{1}{2}$ fl oz)	3
Yogurt, Greek ewe's, per 100 ml (3$\frac{1}{2}$ fl oz)	2
Yogurt, natural low-fat, per 100 ml (3$\frac{1}{2}$ fl oz)	1
Yogurt, whole milk, per 100 ml (3$\frac{1}{2}$ fl oz)	3
Fromage frais, diet fruit, per tub	1
Fromage frais, natural, 0% fat, per 100 ml (3 $\frac{1}{2}$ fl oz)	1
Fromage frais, natural, 8% fat, per 100 ml (3$\frac{1}{2}$ fl oz)	2$\frac{1}{2}$

VEGETABLE PROTEINS

	No. of triangles
Quorn, per 100 g (3¹/₂ oz)	1¹/₂
Tofu, per 100 g (3¹/₂ oz)	1¹/₂
TVP (soya mince), per 100 g (3¹/₂ oz), reconstituted weight	1¹/₂

Group 4: Fats

FATS AND OILS

All per 25 g (1 oz) unless otherwise stated

Butter	4
Margarine	4
Polyunsaturated margarine	4
Low-fat spread	2
Very low-fat spread	1¹/₂
Oil, all types	5
Oil, 1 tablespoon	2¹/₂

DRESSINGS

All per tablespoon (15 ml, ¹/₂ fl oz)

French dressing	2
Mayonnaise	2
Mayonnaise, reduced-calorie	1
Salad cream	1

CHEESES

All per 25 g (1 oz)

Mature Cheddar	2
Cream cheese, full-fat	2¹/₂
Stilton	2¹/₂
Blue Brie	2¹/₂

CREAM AND MILK

	No. of triangles
Single, per 25 ml (1 fl oz)	1
Double, per 25 ml (1 fl oz)	2
Double, half-fat, per 25 ml (1 fl oz)	1
Whipped, per tablespoon	1
Milk, whole, per 75 ml (3 fl oz)	1
Milk, whole, per average glass	3½

FRIED FOODS

Egg size 3, fried, one,	3
Fish, deep-fried in batter, one average portion	6–8
Chips, per 100 g (3½ oz)	5
Oven chips, per 100 g (3½ oz)	3½

MEAT

Bacon, back, average grilled, one slice	3
Bacon, back, trimmed, grilled, one slice	2
Bacon, streaky, grilled, one slice	3
Beef, average minced, per 100 g (3½ oz)	5
Duck, roast, including skin, per 100 g (3½ oz)	7
Lamb shoulder, roast, per 100 g (3½ oz)	6
Lamb chop, including fat, one average	7
Liver sausage, per 50 g (2 oz)	3
Luncheon meat, per 50 g (2 oz)	3
Salami, per 50 g (2 oz)	5
Sausages, beef or pork, grilled, one large	2½
Frankfurter, one	1
Tongue, per 50 g (2 oz)	2

NUTS AND SNACKS

No. of triangles

All per 25 g (1 oz) shelled weight

Almonds or brazils	3
Hazelnuts	2
Peanuts or peanut butter	3
Walnuts	2¹/₂
Crisps, standard	2¹/₂
Crisps, lower fat	2

PASTRY ITEMS

Filo pastry, per 25 g (1 oz)	1¹/₂
Flaky pastry, per 25 g (1 oz)	3
Shortcrust pastry, per 25 g (1 oz)	2¹/₂
Meat pie, one individual	10
Pasty, Cornish, one	9
Pork pie, one individual, 140 g (5 oz)	11

Group 5: Sugars and sweet items

BISCUITS, CONFECTIONERY AND SOFT DRINKS

Biscuits, digestive, each	1¹/₂
Biscuits, chocolate, each	2
Cake, fruit, 50 g (2 oz) slice	3
Cake, sponge, 50 g (2 oz) slice	3
Cheesecake, 75 g (3 oz) slice	6
Chocolate, milk or plain, per 25 g (1 oz)	3
Cola, one can	2¹/₂
Croissant, one small	3
Doughnut, jam, one	4¹/₂

	No. of triangles
Eclair, chocolate, one	3
Fruit pie, 125 g (4½ oz) portion	7
Ice cream, 50 g (2 oz) portion	2
Jam or honey, two teaspoons	1
Lemonade, one can	2
Pastry, Danish, one	7
Sugar, any kind, one teaspoon	½
Sweets, boiled, per 25 g (1 oz)	2
Toffees, per 25 g (1 oz)	2

Group 6: Alcohol

Beer, per 275 ml (½ pint)	2
Lager, per 275 ml (½ pint)	2
Extra-strong lager, per 275 ml (½ pint)	3
Spirits, all, one measure	1
Stout, per 275 ml (½ pint)	2
Wine, medium or dry, 140 ml (5 fl oz) glass	2
Wine, sweet, 140 ml (5 fl oz) glass	3
Champagne, 140 ml (5 fl oz) glass	3